Trees, Healing, and You

Guided Imagery, Poems, Stories, & Other Empowering Tools

by

Kimberly Burnham
Céline Cloutier
Daniel Tigner
Margo Royce
Basia Alexander
Jim Conroy

Trees, Healing, and You
Guided Imagery, Poems, Stories, & Other
Empowering Tools

Cover photo, "Meditation in Old Growth Forest," photo courtesy Daniel Tigner ©2016.

Creating Calm Network Publishing Group
Health / Healing / Nature / Trees

Paperback ISBN: 978-1-937207-19-9

Table of Contents

8

"We travel the Milky Way together, Trees and Men."
—John Muir, *The Dying of the Trees*

"Etherically, trees feed the subtle body of a person. The primary thing it feeds is love."
—Marcel Vogel, *Secrets from the Lives of Trees*

"The creation of a thousand forests is in one acorn."
—Ralph Waldo Emerson

"Don't be ashamed to weep; 'tis right to grieve. Tears are only water, and flowers, trees, and fruit cannot grow without water. But there must be sunlight also. A wounded heart will heal in time, and when it does, the memory and love of our lost ones is sealed inside to comfort us."
—Brian Jacques, *Taggerung*

"The clearest way into the Universe is through a forest wilderness."
—John Muir

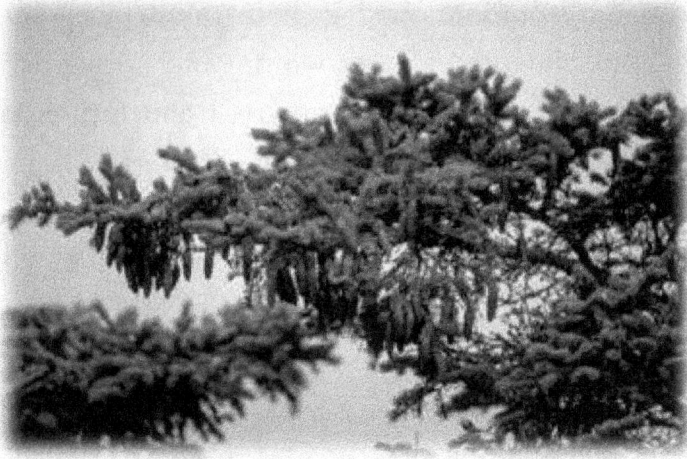

Introduction

Think about the trees around you, at home, at work, and in the places you seek solace or entertainment. Are you enjoying the benefits of the natural world to create physical health and inner peace?

The more one is able to take in the energy, sights, sounds, and vibrations of the world, the easier it is to see the opportunities for healing and connection. Designed to support your health and your ability to connect with trees, the authors: Kimberly Burnham, Céline Cloutier (Gulabo), Daniel Tigner (Hafiz), Margo Royce, Basia Alexander, and Jim Conroy, provide you with exercises to be done in

15

the natural outdoors and in your mind. They share ways to time travel backwards and forwards to connect with the trees of your past and future, and explain how to use poetry, meditation, and visualizations to create colorful and vivid images of the world around you in your mind and in your reality.

Read through the steps. Decide whether you feel comfortable doing these exercises. If you do not feel comfortable with a particular exercise or have any concern whatsoever, do not do it.

You may enjoy these exercises regularly. Making notes each time you do an exercise will give you a sense of your progress.

Here begins a lifelong journey of healing through Traditional Chinese Medicine, Guided Imagery, Meditation, Tree Whispering, and the Poetry of Trees.

— Kimberly Burnham, Editor
2016, Spokane, Washington

"When you have seen one ant, one bird, one tree, you have not seen them all."
—E. O. Wilson

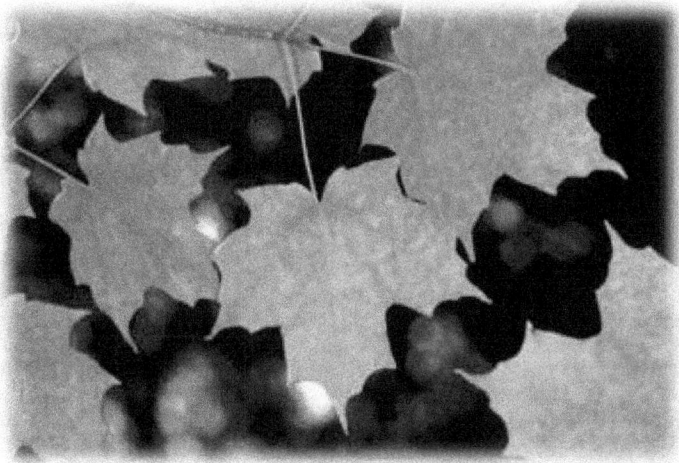

Chapter 1: The Sense of Self

Daniel Tigner (Hafiz)

What is your sense of self? Who are you? Who are you in relationship to the people around you? Who are you in relationship to the environment within which you live? Who are you?

Use the guided imagery in these meditations from Daniel Tigner to develop your sense of self and relationships to others.

Meditation #1 The "Sense of I Am"

Can we truly get to know a tree, even be its friend? And, can a tree get to know us?

We want to explore that question, not as a philosophical discussion, but through hands on exercise and practices that we can learn. What we want is to come to know through our own experience. How do we know anyone or anything? Let's start with knowing our self. If right now, we were to ask ourselves the basic and essential question, *"Who am I?"* where would we arrive?

Come in this moment to a *Sense of I Am* reading these words. Notice that there is an awareness that is aware of all events, perceptions, thoughts and emotions happening in you. You might say *"I am happy or sad."* Feel the *Sense of I Am* on one side and the feeling of being happy or sad on the other side. This a simple awareness exercise which is at the core of meditation practices. Do this practical exercise in awareness as often and whenever you like to come back to yourself.

Notice another quality of awareness: the *Sense of I* is ongoing. That's why you might say, *"When I was a child or I will in the future."* So, the *Sense of I Am* is a constant, underlying all. On the other hand, all objects of perception are constantly changing including your emotions, thoughts, sensations, the body, and the world around you.

Notice also that which you are noticing is always partial, limited and shifting. You are aware of your hand, then your breathing, then a thought and each of those internal events momentarily seems to fill your awareness…. Each moment shifting, but the *Sense of I Am* remains.

"It is important to recognize the reality of our own direct experiences of nature in the wilderness, in the countryside, in forests, on mountains, by the sea, or wherever we have felt ourselves to be in connection with the greater living world. In its stronger forms, this sense of communion has the force of mystical experience, of illumination, surprise, and joy. But when we return to our everyday lives, we have a strong temptation to dismiss such experience as merely subjective, something that just happened inside us and did not involve any real participation in a life greater than our own. I think we should resist this temptation. Our direct experiences of nature are more real and more direct than mere theories, which go in and out of fashion."
—Rupert Sheldrake, *The Rebirth of Nature*

Meditation #2 Exploring Tree Consciousness

Does a tree also have a *Sense of I Am*, and an awareness that is aware of all that it is experiencing, including you - when you are nearby? To find out, it seems to me we need to begin by exploring our own *Sense of I Am*, and then opening ourselves to the possibility of truly encountering a tree. Can't that effort in itself be profoundly insightful and healing as we connect to a greater sense of wholeness?

"The tree is man's best friend and one of God's noblest creations. How dependent we are upon trees has yet to be fully realized. Only in a vague sort of way can we assess the real contribution that trees make to human existence on this planet. Their functions are legion and their life is interwoven with earth and ether. To the trees we owe the quality of our food, the quantity of our water, and the purity of the very air we breathe."
—Richard St. Barbe Baker, *Green Glory*

"When one tugs at a single thing in nature, he finds it attached to the rest of the world."
—John Muir

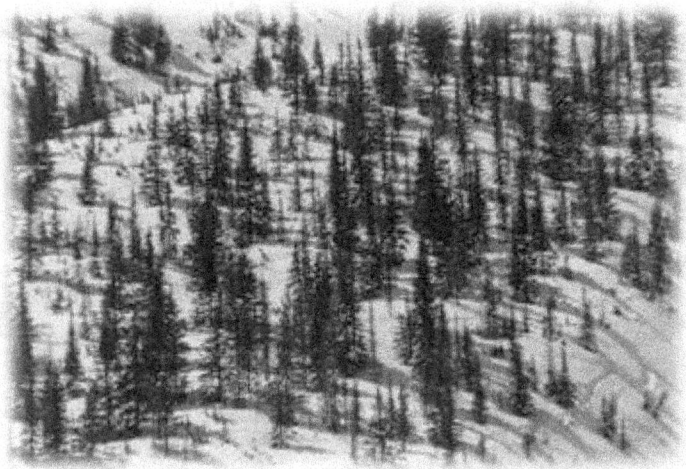

Chapter 2: The Wood Element in Traditional Chinese Medicine

Kimberly Burnham

In Traditional Chinese Medicine, explains Kimberly Burnham, who has a PhD in Integrative Medicine, each organ system is associated with a particular meridian or line of energy in the body. For example, the gallbladder is associated with a line of energy or meridian that travels from the head to the toes along the outside edge of each leg.

Each pair of meridians is also associated with an element and a color. Green is the color connected with the wood elements, which are the liver and gallbladder. The liver meridian travels along the inside of the legs. Pairs of meridians like the liver and gallbladder are also related to particular emotions, tastes, smells, and other sensations as well as influences on brain chemistry.

Here are 12 exercises that help stimulate and balance the Wood Elements and eliminate symptoms associated with these two meridians. Note that the gallbladder and liver are intimately associated with the digestive system and the immune system. On a symbolic level these two organs decide what we take into our body and lives or what we reject.

"Plans to protect air and water, wilderness and wildlife are in fact plans to protect man."
—Stewart Udall

"Conservation is a state of harmony between men and land."
—Aldo Leopold

Exercise #1 A Walking Meditation in the Colors of Nature's Sensational Medicine

Tapping into the benefits of color therapy is a great way to increase the healthy outcomes you get from walking. Here are some things you can do whether you are walking outside in a natural environment or training indoors. Either way consciously paying attention to color can increase your enjoyment of your training sessions and have a positive effect on your vision, brain health, and mood.

In Traditional Chinese Medicine, which includes acupuncture, acupressure, herbs and exercises, practitioners talk about five elements and the colors associated with your organ health and the meridians or lines of energy in your arms and legs.

Here is how you can use this information on your walk.

Noticing the Green of Wood: Green is associated with the Wood elements: the Liver and the Gallbladder.

As you walk pay attention to the color green around you both natural elements and those that are man-made. How many different things can you see that are green? What is the sensation you experience as green hits your eyes?

In Chinese Medicine this kind of attention to your surroundings improves your relationship and connection with your environment and in so doing is thought to improve your liver and gallbladder health.

Another way to look at this is to notice, and this is often very subtle, how your choice of clothing influences how you feel as you walk. At the end of a walk do you feel better if you wear a green shirt or a yellow one? Is there a difference? Often the feelings can be different on different days. What influence do you feel if the color of your shorts or pants, which cover your legs and the liver and gallbladder meridians that run along the inner (liver) and outer side (gallbladder) of each leg, is green? Consciously check in with yourself as you dress for your next walk and see what colors appeal to you the most.

Consider the texture or material that you are seeing as you walk. How many different kinds of trees or plants can you see? Notice how a tree is not all the same color or texture. Notice the roughness of the bark and the different shades of green, white, brown, and black in one small area of a tree.

"Problems cannot be solved at the same level of awareness that created them."
—Albert Einstein

Exercise #2 Enhancing Growth and Vitality

The wood elements are also associated with growth and vitality. Look around as you walk. What do you see that represents growth and vitality to you? Are those things green or some other color?

If you want to bring more growth and vitality into your liver, your gallbladder, or your life, pay attention to the color green. You may be wondering if this works even if you have had your gallbladder removed. Sensational Medicine, noticing the healing benefits of your sensations, is about energy so it works whether you have gallbladder or not.

"The essential core, the spirit of meditation is to learn how to witness. You are seeing a tree: You are there, the tree is there, but can't you find one thing more? — that you are seeing the tree, that there is a witness in you which is seeing you seeing the tree.

The world is not divided only into the object and the subject. There is also something beyond both, and that beyond is meditation."
—Osho

Exercise #3 Metal Fueling Muscles

The Metal elements: Lungs and Large Intestine are associated with the color white and silver.

For exercise, these are key organs as the lungs bring in oxygen to fuel your muscles and large intestine health influences the mobility of the hips and pelvis. These two meridians run along the inner and outer edges of your arms.

As you walk does it change anything if you visualize a flow of white energy from your lungs to your finger tips? Let the white light circulate around your core, chest and abdomen before fueling your legs with power.

The metal elements are also associated with clarity and precision. Focus for a few minutes on the precision of your steps and the evenness of the stride. If you breathe a little deeper in and out are you able to focus with more clarity on your movements?

Take a deep breath. Breathe in the oxygen provided by trees and plants.

"I love the sound of the trees in the breeze. If the forest is so clearly musical, why can't it play the guitar while I sing Nirvana covers?"
— Jarod Kintz, *This Book is Not FOR SALE*

Exercise #4 Yellow Earth Speeding Recovery

The stomach, spleen, and pancreas are the yellow earth elements. What do you see in your environment that is yellow? The Earth elements are also associated with three organ system: the lymphatic system, the digestive system and the muscle system.

Each is vital. The flow through the lymph system allows us to recover from injuries more quickly, decreasing swelling and inflammation after an injury. The digestive system, of course, provides nutrients to fuel our activity, while our muscles allow us to move and create in the world.

Specifically associated with the Earth elements are two muscles, the latissimus dorsi and the pectoralis major. Latissimus dorsi pulls your shoulders back and helps you lift your arm. It is one of the rotator cuff muscles, while pectoralis major pulls the shoulder forward and stabilities the shoulder's ball and socket as you move your arm.

An exercise you can do while standing outside or sitting inside is to place one hand on top of your head and quickly move the opposite shoulder forward and back ten times, then reverse and put the other hand on top of your head. This exercise is designed to cause the muscles of the shoulders to rhythmically contract and relax creating a pumping action that improves the flow of lymph, blood and fluids to and from the head, arms, and body.

Go outside for a few minutes. Notice the way trees grow out of the earth at the interface between the roots and the trunk. Can you ground yourself like a tree in the rich black earth.

"At night I dream that you and I are two plants
that grew together, roots entwined,
and that you know the earth and the rain like my mouth,
since we are made of earth and rain."
—Pablo Neruda, *Regalo de un Poeta*

"Love the trees until their leaves fall off, then encourage
them to try again next year."
—Chad Sugg

"A nation that destroys its soils destroys itself. Forests are
the lungs of our land, purifying the air and giving fresh
strength to our people."
—Franklin D. Roosevelt

Exercise #5 Fiery Red

Red is the color of the fire elements. There are four Fire elements, which are associated with passion and high energy and include the heart, of course, and the pericardium (the connective tissue around and protecting the heart). The small intestine absorbs the fire in your food. What red foods have you eaten today? Apples, pomegranates, and blood oranges are all red tree fruit.

The fourth Fire element is called the Triple Warmer and is not an organ but represents the endocrine and hormone related systems. Working with the fire elements can help with your body's temperature regulation including cold hands and hot flashes.

As you are walking, what do you see that is red? How many shades of red do you see? Red is the easiest to see and the fastest color to reach our eyes, which is why stop signs and brake lights are red.

A healthy fire element system speeds up recovery and slows down degeneration. Visualize the red of iron ore in Red Rock country, oxygen rich red blood cells, a shiny apple, juicy round tomatoes, the reddish tint of organic kale, or a red light turning green. Let the red in your environment nourish your passion.

Exercise #6 The Ease and Abundance of Blue Water

The final element, water is predictably, blue. Imagine the ease and abundance of the flow in a wide river. Now imagine the flow of fluids within your body orchestrated by the kidneys and bladder.

How blue is the sky as you walk? Do you see any blue birds? The people around you, are any of them wearing blue, the color of kidney and bladder healing?

Imagine the color blue circulating through your mid and low back area, the physical location of the kidneys and bladder.

Notice all the colors around you. Look around at the scenery. Are you seeing it differently after consciously considering each of these colors? Are the greens brighter? Do you notice more white objects? How does it feel to look at the yellow earth tones around you? Does the red make you smile? Do you feel calmer just by noticing a blue lake with green trees by it's shore?

Exercise #7 Improving Vision

The gallbladder meridian starts near the eyes and the wood elements (liver and gallbladder) are associated with eye health and the sense of vision.

In a complementary medicine approach known as Emotional Freedom Technique (EFT) or Tapping, the client taps on the eye brow and then the side of the eye as well as other points on the body, while saying a phrase like, *"Even though my vision isn't perfect, I see so much beauty around myself,"* or *"Even though I have a headache, I love and accept myself anyway."*

What would be a good phrase for you? What is going on with your eyes, face or head that you consider a symptom that you want to resolve? At the same time, what can you think of that is positive about your situation in life?

Think of the phrase Even though _____, I _____ .

Walk outside and repeat your phrase several times, while tapping on the eye brow and / or the side of the eye.

Alternatively you can sit quietly inside with your eyes closed and visualize a beautiful forest or woods as you repeat your phrase several times.

Exercise #8 Improving Sleep

This sensory awareness exercise will help you sleep deeper, release eye strain, enjoy more of the beauty around you, and improve peripheral vision

This is also great for people who want to recognize the detail in another person's face and improve relationships.

Use this for relaxation. For people that have trouble sleeping, it's a great exercise to do about a half an hour before you want to go to sleep, just to really get yourself present to your sensations and connected to how you feel.

In this exercise, start by looking around yourself and noticing how you feel. What does your body feel like? What do you notice about your surroundings? Feel your environment. Look at your environment. Notice where you are in time and in space.

Then pick up an item, a relatively small item that you can hold in your hands. Describe it in as sensory terms as possible. What this means is describe the color, the shapes, the size, the texture, the temperature, the sound of it, the taste of it, and the smell of it? Use all your sense to describe it.

What I say to my one-on-one clients is, I should be able to walk in to your house after hearing your description and find the item that you described to me, from your description. I should be able to tell what it is.

For example, I am holding an item. I am going to describe it to you. I am not going to tell you what it is until the end. But, I'm hoping that from my description you will be able to recognize what it is. This item is kind of long and cylindrical and it has a pointy part at one end and a kind of a flat surface at the other end. It is white with kind of a tan design on it and part of the design has small oval shapes. Along the smooth middle part is some writing and the letters are raised a little bit, with a bumpy texture. So, as I run my finger along the writing on this item, I can feel little bumps. There is also a piece at one end opposite the pointy end that is kind of a large oval piece. It is a harder material than the rest of the item. And it is attached by a little ring around the top part of the item. If I tap it, I can hear a sound, that tells me it's a kind of plastic material, and then there is a clicking mechanism that causes the pointy part to go in and out. This doesn't really have a taste. It's not a food item. It doesn't really have a smell. Maybe when it was brand new it might have had a plastic kind of a smell.

And I hope that by now you know that what I had in my hand is a pen, a click pen. That is the kind of detail that I would like you to use to describe. It is best to do it out loud, it doesn't have to be with someone else, but you can call up a friend and say, *"Kim gave me this exercise. Can I just describe an item to you?"*

See if they can guess what the item is from your description of all the different sensations. It doesn't have to be a long time, it can be just a few minutes. Describe something now.

As you noticed it's not just visual information, you're really taking in all the information, through all your five senses. Through your eyes, your ears, and sense of taste and smell, if it has those things. And certainly touch, texture, and shape.

This exercise is even better if you pick up an item made of wood.

"A cold wind was blowing from the north, and it made the trees rustle like living things."
—George R.R. Martin, *A Game of Thrones*

Exercise #9 Healing in Movement Disorders

Do you ever describe yourself as stiff as a board?

Alive a tree is full of growth and vitality. Dead it is stiff as a board. The same is true of your cells. What brings life, growth, and vitality into your cells? Healthy wood elements (liver and gallbladder) contribute to adaptability, flexibility and speedy cellular repair.

The wood elements are also associated with the brain chemical dopamine, which when imbalanced contributes to conditions like Parkinson's disease (stiffness and loss of muscle control) and schizophrenia (loss of connection to reality, the ability to imagine, and to be able to tell the difference).

As you walk outdoors pay attention to your liver and gallbladder. The liver is located on your right side behind the lower rib cage. If you place your right hand so that your little finger is along the lower right border of your rib cage, the rest of your hand will be over the area of your liver. The gallbladder sits behind the liver, along the lower edge in the center. Notice as you rest your hand over the liver area whether it feel the same as the opposite side of the rib cage. Located behind the lower rib cage on the left is the spleen and tail of the pancreas.

Do you ever get a "stitch" in these areas as you exercise? Flexing your back and stretching can help.

As you exercise notice how your back feels. Is there vitality in the area around T9 to T10? T stands for the Thoracic spine. There are 12 thoracic vertebra, each with a rib attached. T9 is the lower end and associated with liver health. T10, just below it is associated with the gallbladder in the acupuncture meridian system.

Move your back a little as you walk or move. Do you have the flexibility you want?

Two muscles are associated with the acupuncture's wood elements (liver and gallbladder) and therefore with the brain chemical dopamine. The anterior deltoid muscle at the shoulder and popliteus at the back of the knee are associated with the gallbladder, while the pectoralis major sternal segment of the chest muscles and rhomboids at the back of the shoulders are associated with the liver.

Notice these areas as you stretch and move. Stretching should always be pain-free. Do not stretch through the pain. Stretch to a comfortable range and then imagine yourself stretching to the end range. Little by little you may find yourself stretching comfortably farther and farther.

What if you just started by imagining yourself doing stretches first thing in the morning or in the evening before you fall asleep. Imagine how your back and shoulders would feel. What changes would there be in the circulation to the big muscles of your arms and legs and to your brain just by imagining yourself stretching?

Here is what researchers say about the use of imagery or meditation and dopamine in the brain.

Imagine what can change and how rewarding just imagining yourself doing these stretch and exercises would be.

"In meditation both the quality and the contents of consciousness may be voluntarily changed, making it an obvious target in the quest for the neural correlate of consciousness. Meditation is accompanied by a relatively increased perfusion [blood flow] in the sensory imagery system [where you imagine sensations]. Our subsequent finding of increased striatal [part of the brain] dopamine binding to D2 receptors during meditation suggested dopaminergic regulation of this [sensory imagery and consciousness] circuit."
—Lou, H. C., M. Nowak, et al. (2005). "The mental self." Prog Brain Res 150: 197-204.

Exercise #10 See The Wood Elements Around You

Another way to support your liver and gallbladder is to see the wood elements in your environment whether you are riding a bicycle outside, training indoors, or walking.

Look around yourself. Notice the variety of green, the Traditional Chinese Medicine color of the wood elements. Notice the shades of green. How would you describe the difference between the green of freshly mowed grass, the leaves on a springtime maple tree, or the pine needles juxtaposed against the reddish bark of a pine tree? How much detail can you see in rough tree bark? Imagine the texture of one tree trunk compared to another. Notice the repeating branching pattern in the trees around you. This is known as a fractal pattern where the big thing is like the small thing only bigger. Even the leaves have a tiny branching central vein similar to the trunk with branches.

And finally, green bile, produced in the liver and stored in the gallbladder helps digest fats in your diet—fats that are needed for the membranes around your muscles, the building of nerves and brain function, and the creation of hormonal balance. Do you have enough "good fats" in your diet? High in "good" fats and iron, cashews, walnuts and other tree nuts can be a good snack while you are exercising.

To see a World in a grain of sand,
And a Heaven in a wild flower,
Hold Infinity in the palm of your hand,
And Eternity in an hour.
—William Bake

"To be poor and be without trees, is to be the most starved
human being in the world. To be poor and have trees, is to
be completely rich in ways that money can never buy."
—Clarissa Pinkola Estés, *The Faithful Gardener: A Wise*
Tale About That Which Can Never Die

"Rilke wrote: 'These trees are magnificent, but even more
magnificent is the sublime and moving space between them,
as though with their growth it too increased."
—Gaston Bachelard, *The Poetics of Space*

"Of all the trees we could've hit, we had to get one that hits
back."
—J.K. Rowling, *Harry Potter and the Chamber of Secrets*

Exercise #11 Detoxifying in the Woods

Another way to use this information is to understand that the liver and gallbladder are organs of detoxification and digestion.

Take a walk in the woods while noticing all the wood and color green around you. Take deep breaths. Take in the smell of the trees around you. Notice the taste of tree fruit.

"I fall in love with you four times a year: winter, spring, summer, and fall. The leaves may change, but how I feel about you does not."
—Jarod Kintz, *This Book is Not FOR SALE*

"I'm planting a tree to teach me to gather strength from my deepest roots."
—Andrea Koehle Jones, *The Wish Trees*

"If you love music, you love it only because around it somehow you feel meditation happening. You are absorbed by it, you become drunk in it. Something of the unknown starts descending in you..."
—Osho, *The Everyday Meditator*

Exercise #12 Anger Management

All of these exercises can also help with anger management because the wood elements (liver and gallbladder) are associated with the emotion of anger in Traditional Chinese Medicine or acupuncture.

The emotions associated with the gallbladder and liver are anger and compassion. Notice how these emotions affect your body and move accordingly. Imagine yourself physically expressing your anger in a constructive way. Imagine yourself in an act of compassion. What is the body posture of compassion?

As you move, imagine yourself as an actor in an improvisation group where you have to act out or express anger or compassion? How would you move differently if you were angry compared to feeling compassion? Does anger ever get in the way of your exercise schedule? Use visualization to help you express and harness rather than suppress these two emotions.

In summary, there are several ways to harness the sensational medicine of the wood elements: notice the wood and trees around you, the color green, how your body feels in the area of the liver and gallbladder, the flexibility in your lower mid-back, and a sense of balance between anger and compassion. It is the act of paying attention that is important and healing.

"Two Trees
A portion of your soul has been
entwined with mine
A gentle kind of togetherness, while
separately we stand.
As two trees deeply rooted in
separate plots of ground,
While their topmost branches
come together,
Forming a miracle of lace
against the heavens."
—Janet Mills, *The Power of a Woman*

"Standing as the earth's largest and oldest living monuments, I believe these symbolic trees will take on a greater significance, especially at a time when our focus is directed at finding better ways to live with the environment"
—Beth Moon, a photographer based in San Francisco, searches for the world's oldest trees, capturing the most magnificent trees that grow in remote locations and look as old as the world itself.

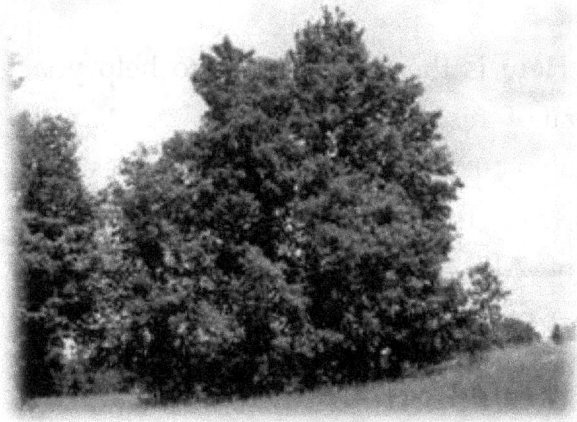

Chapter 3: Making a Nature Connection

Basia Alexander and Jim Conroy

Dr. Jim Conroy, PhD, The Tree Whisperer® and Ms. Basia Alexander, offer seven exercises for making a deeply intuitive and spiritually profound connection with Nature. As an added bonus, comments and tips from their Tree Whispering students illuminate important points.

Exercise #1 Know Yourself

Here is the first exercise to help you get the most out of this book.

If you love trees, plants, forests, and the planet—and have hope for a positive future—then check off ALL the reasons why you were attracted to the idea of healing through trees and to the idea of communicating with nature for mutual healing.

___ I love trees and plants. I am a "plant person."

___ I already talk to trees and plants.

___ They talk to me, too.

___ It sounded interesting and I enjoy learning new things.

___ I want to know that I'm not alone; there are other people like me.

___ I want to be inspired.

___ I want to be more creative.

___ I want to heal my body.

___ I want to become more intuitive.

___ I'm curious.

___ I want to get closer to nature.

___ I want to awaken the perceptions I had as a child.

____ I enjoy feeling good (healing in body and soul) when I am with plants or trees.

____ I think this might be rejuvenating for me.

____ I am concerned about the health of a certain tree in my yard.

____ I want to save an historic tree.

____ I believe I can help sick trees; I want to do "good" for another living being.

____ I want to care for my trees or plants without chemicals or invasive techniques.

____ I want to preserve my investment in my home's landscape.

____ I am a tree professional and want to explore something new.

____ I want to grow a better garden or do better at farming.

____ I am grateful for all that trees and plants give me.

____ Trees have taught me about life.

____ I have good memories of trees.

____ I am concerned about the environment and the planet and want to help the trees, plants, crops, and forests in some way.

____ I suspect that this fits into my expanding view of life and the global paradigm shift in consciousness that is going on now.

____ Other: _____

Exercise #2 Validate Yourself

People who hear about the idea of communicating with nature beings, often approach us, Dr. Jim and Basia, and describe a feeling of relief in realizing that their childhood perceptions or adult encounters with Nature Beings were authentic and credible. Some share with us that they talk to plants secretly but now are inspired to accept the truth of their experiences and share with others.

Sometimes people unfairly judge themselves. They may have been influenced by historical or cultural biases concerning their character and intelligence. We encourage all to approve of and accept themselves.

Here are some ways to validate yourself.

1. Know and tell your own truth.

2. Give yourself permission to be as you are, not as someone else wants you to be.

3. Forgive yourself for a perceived transgression.

4. Examine existing beliefs, then author new and more supportive beliefs.

5. Say "yes" to yourself.

6. Praise or acknowledge your own qualities.

7. Accept that your behavior is authentic to your inner inspiration.

8. Take actions based on your beliefs.

9. Be confident and persistent, even in the face of disagreement.

Our workshop graduates have shared their thoughts with us:

Leslie, project manager: ... *"I knew that the inklings and intuitions I had previously in my life were true. But, more than that, I knew I was feeling the right things. There were no questions inside of me. Being sure about my own perceptions opened up changes and new freedom in my life."*

Lori, office manager and energy medicine practitioner: *"Sometimes I feel that trees say funny things to me and that gives me great joy. On one occasion, I felt someone walking down the path and seeing me giggling with a tree. I said to myself, "Oh well, it's silly to be self-conscious." I realized that it didn't matter to me whether anyone saw me or what they thought of me."*

Debra, wellness director for an international children's art project: *"As a child, if I were upset, I would go to my favorite tree and feel better. I also wrote poetry while sitting beneath its branches. I seemed to get phrases; ideas would just pop in. Now, I'm sure that the tree was helping me. If you have a favorite tree from childhood, I recommend that you return to it. Perhaps you can reclaim some of your childhood wonder. It may be happy to see you again and give you fresh insights and inspiration."*

Connecting With Living Systems

Trees are family. Not 'like' family, they are family. And, so are insects, creatures in the soil, animals, fungi, bees, reptiles, all kinds of microorganisms including disease organisms, and even those living beings we call "invasives." All living beings are children of the same mother: Earth.

All have a kind of consciousness, whether some people think they do or not. To have physical form means that a spiritual energy or a consciousness has elected to express itself in a body of some kind. At least, believing that is true works for me.

Where there is cognition there is an intelligence that can share information. With consciousness at the foundation of all life, communication is possible. All living beings can connect—like to like and unlike to unlike.

Please see the reading list at the end of this book for scientific and other references.

"If you really want to eat, keep climbing. The fruits are on the top of the tree. Stretch your hands and keep stretching them. Success is on the top, keep going."
—Israelmore Ayivor

Exercise #3 A Quiet Walk in the Woods

Don't you feel good—body and soul—when you feel connected with nature? You leave behind your cares when you immerse yourself in the pleasures of the fragrance of pine needles or the rustle of a deep green canopy of leaves in the breeze. Perhaps on a quiet walk in the woods, you think that—for a moment—you are leaving your world and step into the trees' world.

Read through the steps of this exercise. If you do not feel comfortable or have any concern whatsoever, do not do it.

1. Go to your favorite park, woods, forest, or path through trees.

2. Begin your walk in a quiet, peaceful state.

3. In your heart or speaking in a whisper, express gratitude to the trees as you move among them. You may say things such as, *"I am grateful for your life. I appreciate your beauty. Thank you for your gifts."*

4. Notice how you feel when you offer these acknowledgements.

5. Stop for a moment. Say to the trees: *"I open my heart to you."* Then wait, focus on your feelings, listen with your inner ears, and see with your inner eyes.

6. Resume walking. Be receptive to feelings or the messages coming to you from them.

7. As you walk or afterward, jot down notes about how you feel, what you think, and what it was like for you to take this walk. Writing brief phrases is okay.

"If lightning is the anger of the gods, then the gods are concerned mostly about trees."
—Lao Tzu

"Trees are poems that the earth writes upon the sky."
—Khalil Gibran, *Sand and Foam*

"Why are there trees I never walk under but large and melodious thoughts descend upon me?"
—Walt Whitman

"I want to be magic. I want to touch the heart of the world and make it smile. I want to be a friend of elves and live in a tree. Or under a hill. I want to marry a moonbeam and hear the stars sing. I don't want to pretend at magic anymore. I want to be magic."
—Charles de Lint

Exercise #4 Feeling the Heart's Bioenergy Field

People's most sensitive and powerful organ of perception is the heart. The human heart is like another brain. It is made of neural tissue. It also broadcasts and receives signal in the form of a bioenergy field. Think of using a cellular phone. It has a power source. It is connected to the network through an invisible electromagnetic signal so voice goes out and voice comes in. Every living being has an inner power source and is connected to the network of life through an invisible electromagnetic field sometimes called the "bioenergy field."

At the HeartMath Institute, researchers have measured the bioenergy field of the human heart in a vortex shape outside the physical body. Their research has also shown that when two people are either touching or just close to each other, their heart fields overlap so that a physical synchronization of their heartbeats may result. The overlap of bioenergy fields between people is real—it's often how people know if they like another person or not.

"To thine own self be true," said Shakespeare. This means knowing your own heart. What better place to start than being aware of the bioenergy field that your heart generates?

Here are some ways to create awareness of your heart field. Read through the steps. Decide whether you feel comfortable doing this exercise. This and other exercises are available as MP3s.

1. Sit down in a comfortable and private place where you won't be interrupted for about ten minutes. This exercise may be done with eyes closed, if you are comfortable.

2. You have a donut-shaped bioenergy field around you. Pause for a moment and allow yourself to experience your own bioenergy field radiating from your heart.

3. Imagine that you can see your bioenergy field's shape or feel its warmth.

4. Play with your bioenergy field. Ask it to expand, then contract, like the beating heart from which it comes. Respect the field by allowing this to occur. Do not try to force it. Simply ask for expansion and contraction, then watch it happen for as long as is comfortable for you.

5. Think about what having a bioenergy field generated by your heart means to you.

6. Think about the fact that bioenergy fields can overlap. What does that mean to you?

7. Jot down a few notes about your experience. If necessary, sit quietly with your pen poised on the paper. Just to get the pen moving, try writing some

pleasant words such as "beating heart, glowing sun, expansion, contraction, or love."

"Man has to reconsider all traditions, all different sources, whatever facts have become available have to be reconsidered. A totally new medical approach has to be evolved which takes note of acupuncture, which takes note of ayurveda, which takes note of Greek medicine, which takes note of Delgado and his Researches—which takes note of the fact that man is not a machine. Man is a multidimensional spiritual being, and you should behave with him in the same way."
—Osho, *From Medication to Meditation*

"I felt my lungs inflate with the onrush of scenery—air, mountains, trees, people. I thought, 'This is what it is to be happy."
—Sylvia Plath, *The Bell Jar*

"You are a child of the universe, no less than the trees and the stars. In the noisy confusion of life, keep peace in your soul."
—Max Ehrmann

Exchange Information with Other Living Beings

It makes sense that other living beings would also generate bioenergy fields. This invisible overlapping exchange of electromagnetic field energy is how ecosystem members have been sharing information—communicating—with each other throughout their billions of years of evolutionary development on Earth. Such an *invisible yet real* exchange of messages occurs everywhere in nature over and above physical exchanges such as roots touching, chemical emissions, clicks, howls, or human speech.

So, it is up to people—yes, you and me—to shift our mindsets and expand our capacities for communication so that the other living, intelligent, conscious beings on Earth can get their important messages through to us.

"A tree against the sky possesses the same interest, the same character, the same expression as the figure of a human."
—Georges Rouault

Exercise #5 Shifting Mindsets

Here is an opportunity to take an inventory of some of the notions that you may still contain concerning your ability to communicate with nature beings and then shift those toward what feels better and what you want. These would be the ideas, attitudes, or beliefs that you picked up in the general culture, from your family, or from schooling that are limiting you in some way. Don't dwell on what is negative, just become aware of phrases that surface for you.

Once you have a few of those, you want to change them into something that *feels better*. It has to feel good; it doesn't have to be the opposite idea. Don't stretch too far to where the idea doesn't seem real or doesn't make sense to you; just move onto the next thought that feels better.

On the left side of a sheet of paper, write down a few ideas, attitudes, or beliefs that are limiting to you in some way about having mutual communication with the living beings of nature. Then, for each entry on the left, on the right write down the next good feeling thought. Continue on another piece of paper if necessary.

Moving toward the next better feeling or thought is the beginning of shifting your mindset from old, self-limiting notions into a new world of freedom, capability, and possibility for yourself. This exercise can be done about any topic.

Every person will have a different experience. All who want to communicate with the beings of nature can do so by becoming better receivers. Developing keen perception with the physical senses and opening to emotional receptivity both contribute to expanded intuition.

"The planting of a tree, especially one of the long-living hardwood trees, is a gift which you can make to posterity at almost no cost and with almost no trouble, and if the tree takes root it will far outlive the visible effect of any of your other actions, good or evil."
—George Orwell

"Tree planting is always a utopian enterprise, it seems to me, a wager on a future the planter doesn't necessarily expect to witness."
—Michael Pollan, *Second Nature: A Gardener's Education*

Exercise #6 Sensory Sensitivity

Why is sensory sensitivity so important? Our physical and subtle senses are how we know the world. Tuning them up—like turning up the volume—will help you be more aware of the indirect ways that beings, who do not have language or faces, must use in order to get their messages to us. Messages from trees, plants, and others often come through visualizations or symbols, tingles in the skin, words that come into the inner hearing, and even through fragrance.

1. Touch: physical sensation, gut feeling, knowing at a distance

2. Sight: visual perception or envisioning, visualizing, having imagery

3. Hearing: auditory perception, listening to the inner voice

4. Smell: perceiving fragrance, discovery, clarity

5. Taste: perceiving flavor, sensitivity, discernment

The exercise uses breathing and gentle tapping on the body to provide the conditions in which the body and mind can enhance sensory sensitivity. Your heart area is in the center of your chest, under the sternum, not where you hold your hand for the pledge of allegiance. Tap gently at the center of the chest with the fingertips of both hands. Tapping there for the duration of two or three breaths engages the heart-brain so that it will apply its leadership to all the cells of the body through heart beat and blood movement.

Tapping on the skull is like telling the head-brain to awaken to a change that is coming. Tap on both sides of the centerline of the skull gently with fingertips of both hands. You may tap anywhere from your forehead to the top of your head, to the back, just so long as you tap on both sides.

You may or may not feel an immediate enhancement of the chosen sense. The exercise will not enhance the chosen sense by itself. The sense will be enhanced however by repeated focus on any thought, feeling, or idea which tends to expand it.

1. Sit down in a comfortable and private place where you won't be interrupted for about ten minutes. This exercise is best done with eyes closed.

2. Choose one single sense, possibly from the list above that you want to enhance. You can always return to this exercise and enhance another sense.

3. Focus on the sense and take comfortable, deep breaths. Think thoughts that feel good about what you will do with this enhanced sense. If you feel stressed about this, think more general, non-specific thoughts or stop. Do not do anything that is uncomfortable for you.

4. Gently tap with the fingertips of both hands on the heart (center of the chest). Continue to take three or four comfortable breaths while you tap on the heart and focus on the sense and how good you feel.

5. Gently tap with the fingertips of both hands, each on opposite sides of the head. You may tap anywhere: front, top, back, or sides. Do this while taking three to four comfortable breaths. Focus on the sense and how good you feel.

6. Repeat steps four and five several times while focusing your attention on the sense and on how good you feel.

7. Open your eyes, breathe gently, and sit quietly for a moment.

8. Jot down any comments or reflections.

The secrets are in the plants. To elicit them you have to love them enough.
—George Washington Carver, 19th Century Agricultural Chemist, *The Secret Life of Plants*

"Anything else you're interested in is not going to happen if you can't breathe the air and drink the water. Don't sit this one out. Do something."
—Carl Sagan

Trust Intuitive Perception of Messages From Nature

What is intuition? The dictionary definition of the noun is: direct perception of truth, fact, etc., independent of any reasoning process, immediate apprehension, or a keen and quick insight, an immediate cognition of an object not inferred or determined by a previous cognition of the same object pure, untaught, non-inferential knowledge

So, in simpler words, an intuition is a message that comes into your awareness.

Everyone has the capacity to be highly intuitive. Here's advice from graduates of Tree Whispering® workshops for opening yourself, trusting intuition, and being a better receiver of messages from Nature's living Beings.

Cheryl, PhD., Plant Pathology, university extension professor: *"I think a lot of people are hesitant to believe they can receive messages from trees. They wonder, "Am I putting my own thoughts in?" I would advise you to slow down, allow your own Spirit and your energy some freedom. Believe in your energy and the path it may take. It will only give you more energy and freedom. Don't be embarrassed. Welcome the gift of the moment."*

Lori, energy therapy practitioner: *"I suggest that people go out, sit under a tree, breathe and relax, listen* and feel. Most importantly, be patient. Let thoughts come and go; be quiet. Try touching the tree–touching helps in the beginning. Pick one tree and visit it often. It will feel more familiar each time. Simply have fun, be playful!"

Alana, massage therapist and healer: "I try to feel like I am talking on the phone: a connection gets made and I hear the tree or plant speak."

Sylvia, graphic designer and homeowner: "Keep an open mind. Have no distractions. Your "now" presence is required to be with nature. Be mindful of where your focus is directed."

Madeline, business owner and counselor: "Your intuitive sense uses imagination; it uses specific metaphors that you—and only you—are going to understand; it uses the concepts to which you already personally relate. In this way, the intuitive sense aims you toward the information you will need. At the same time, it's important for you to have good, personal boundaries. You need to know what to allow into your body, mind, and spirit. Be discerning."

Judy, artist and landowner: "I go up to a tree to meet it. Within minutes, I can feel the tree's energy, usually in my heart or solar plexus and sometimes I feel a pulsing in my hands. Painting has also been a great way to develop a connection to nature."

Rocky, businessman: "I have expanded my perceptions by being totally open and nonjudgmental. I do this by not expecting myself to get a certain thing. You can't judge a book by its cover; you can't tell what is going on for a being on the inside by what you see on the outside only. So I realized that I had to be forgiving about getting messages from the trees. The best way to get better at perception is do it more often. I play the trumpet. Even though I know what notes to press, if I don't play often, my lip muscles aren't strong. Practicing builds up the perception."

Joan, gardener and homeowner: "Be aware of what's happening as you go for a walk in the woods. Pay attention beyond the little circle just around you. When you are with a plant, tell it what you appreciate about it."

Mary, attorney: "It seems to me that our biggest stumbling block is self-doubt. We have a great capability to negate our innate intuitive abilities. We have also tuned out [our senses] in order to manage in this fast-paced world. But, I think that when we approach Nature with the intent to ask it about itself, feelings and words will come forth. And, if we do it enough, then the doubt is eliminated."

Jeff, horticulturalist: "Developing the heart space is the most important — the heart is a perceptive tool. Using the mind only, I wouldn't have the ability to reach deep into Nature. The best information does not come through thoughts and mind; it comes through feelings. My advice is to recognize the consciousness in Nature."

Cathy, acupuncturist and herbalist: *"Trust that it is our gift and our birthright as humans to be able to communicate with trees and plants. The ability is within all of us."*

Gerry, arborist: *"It's about receptivity—allowing something to come and allowing something good to be given back. I use a little secret to expand my trust in my heart. I tap on the center of my chest while I give my heart's energy-center permission to be and permission to have its own say. Then, I tap between my eyebrows and tell my heart's energy to be uppermost while it links with my head-brain. I do this tapping back and forth from heart-brain to head-brain many times, asking them to work in conjunction. It helps me settle down."*

Georgette, postal worker and homeowner: *"Trust that you didn't make it up. I figure if you get impressions from people when you meet them, why not get an impression from a tree when you meet it? Believing in my impressions was validated for me during a workshop I took. The hotel lobby had an island of tropical plants. I remember that I had the impression that the tall palms didn't want us to touch them because–all day long–people brush by them without thinking or saying "Excuse me." Later, another student and I compared notes and discovered that we both had the same impression!"*

Danielle, newspaper columnist: *"I used to resist, but now I accept perceptions as they come. I simply* recognize the fear and get past it. When I let go, the limiting things I believe go away. I allow what I feel to come to me and accept that it is okay, that it is right."

Chucky, arborist: "I used to get clearer messages as a young person. Now it seems that if a message doesn't show up on a flaming billboard, then I think I'm not getting it. I have criticized myself for losing touch, but I realized that people change and, so, forgive myself. I know that all I need is a little practice."

Liz, copy editor: "We all have those thoughts, wondering if we are crazy or wondering what others will think of us. It's natural. But you want to distract yourself from the inner chatter and just receive the experience and record it while it is happening, writing it down will distract the ego part of the mind from the wonderful flow of direct information that is happening. So, I say to you, "Trust your first impression always." I suggest that you bring a notebook and pens or pencils when you connect with the energy of trees and plants. You should record the messages you get immediately. If you are receiving words, write them. If you are inspired to draw, then draw."

Robin, author, herbalist, and teacher: "Sharing breath is the best starting point. Be as quiet in the mind as possible and open your heart. Let go of the desire for anything in particular to happen. You can imagine a figure-8 of breath and energy going back and forth between you and the tree."

Exercise #7 Make an Intuitive Connection and Get a Message

This is an exercise with a figure-8 of breath and energy going between you and a tree in order to get a message from that nature being.

You should be receiving positive information and pleasant sensations, not pain or discomfort of any kind. If you feel pain inside your body, stop the process immediately. Develop strong, healthy personal and psychological boundaries before you connect with and work with a tree, plant, or other being. Use good, common sense to take care of yourself.

Preparation: Make sure you are in a pleasant and private place where you won't be interrupted for 15-20 minutes.

There will be times during the exercise that you may want to close your eyes, if you are comfortable doing that. Do this exercise standing or sitting outside privately with a tree. Or, you may be indoors and have a plant near you that you can touch. Have your notebook or journal handy to write down some notes about your experiences. It's best to make notes immediately in case you don't remember later.

1. Go to a tree or plant, and put your hands on the tree or plant.

2. Imagine a stream of air coming into your heart area from the tree and going out your belly area back to the tree. This stream of air creates a connection cycle.

3. On the incoming stream of air, imagine the Life Force and bioenergy of the tree connecting with you.

4. On the outgoing stream of air, imagine your Life Force and bioenergy connecting with the tree.

5. Continue to make the cycle of connection for a few minutes: the tree's Life Force is coming in at your heart area and your Life Force is going to the tree from your belly area. It's a mutual exchange of caring or love.

6. Imagine that the tree is a transmitting tower. Imagine that it is sending out something like radio waves in all directions.

7. Imagine that you are a radio receiver. Imagine that you can tune to the station and receive the tree's waves.

8. Imagine the reverse. You are a transmitting tower and the tree is a radio receiver, receiving your waves.

9. Imagine that the tree and you are making a circular, two-way, transmitting-and-receiving cycle.

10. Open your awareness to any message that the tree might be transmitting to you. Then, transmit a message of kindness or love to the tree.

11. Breathe in and out easily and gently. Allow yourself to enjoy this cycle for several minutes. Thank the tree for making the connection with you.

12. Write down a few brief phrases to remind you of your experience. Let the words flow from your heart.

i thank You God for most this amazing
day: for the leaping greenly spirits of trees
and a blue true dream of sky; and for everything
which is natural which is infinite which is yes
(i who have died am alive again today,
and this is the sun's birthday; this is the birth
day of life and of love and wings: and of the gay
great happening illimitably earth)
how should tasting touching hearing seeing
breathing any-lifted from the no
of all nothing-human merely being
doubt unimaginably You?
(now the ears of my ears awake and
now the eyes of my eyes are opened)
— e.e. Cummings

On deforestation ... "Trees, how many of 'em do we need to look at?"
—Ronald Reagan

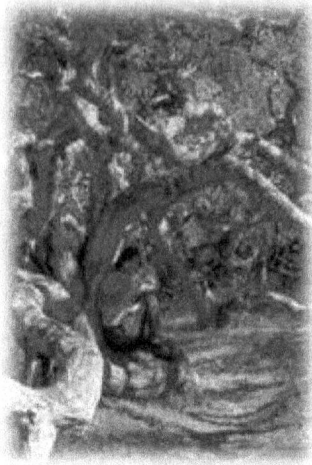

Chapter 4: The Tree Whisperer's Stories of Messages from Trees

Jim Conroy and Basia Alexander

Dr. Jim Conroy tells this story: The question always comes up: Which tree in a community of trees do I pick to treat with my bioenergy-based hands-on, tree-healing process? It is the tree that calls out to me. How does it call? For me, it is a matter of tuning my inner receiver to hear the messages that trees are broadcasting.

The owner of a small and young Apple orchard in Iowa showed me a particular sick tree and expected me to treat that tree. But, my inner antenna was picking up *"help me"* from another tree. The owner was confused. I replied, *"But this one is calling—and they will all receive my bioenergy treatment because they are connected in community."*

As I started to do my healing work on the tree that called out to me, I bent down low to the ground to touch the soil area. My hands were near the base of the trunk. As I touched the area, I felt something under my fingers. I pushed back the turf and soil. There it was: a nylon rope starting to strangle the tree. The rope was a support when the tree was originally planted a few years back. It had slipped down and was now very tight because the trunk had grown. It would have killed the tree by cutting into its cambium layer and stopping movement of fluids.

The owner jumped up and ran to the house to get a knife. We cut the rope, feeling great relief. Then, I heard the tree convey, *"Thank you."*

In 2011, there was a severe late October snowstorm on the East Coast of the USA. People called it the Halloween Storm, and it was scary. Trees were still wearing most of their leaves at the time the storm hit, so countless limbs were lost.

A homeowner called the following April with concerns about a clump of River Birches. Their tops snapped off. They lost many side limbs, too. When I connected with the Birch trees, they told me that the branches they lost were important to their food production capacity. It's important to remember that trees and plants make their own food in their leaves. The loss of so much leaf-surface meant they would have less energy available.

River Birches in Randolph, NJ gave this message: *"We need to produce enough food to sustain ourselves and put on new growth. If our systems are efficient, we need less food-energy to sustain ourselves. Since we lost potential leaves in the storm, we lost some food-making capacity that would help us make new growth. New growth means more leaves which means more food, which means more growth. Then the cycle can continue."*

"Help us make our processes more efficient. With more efficient inner processes, that means less energy needed to sustain us and more energy available for our purpose, which is to grow. More energy available means more new growth and more health for us."

I opened my heart to overlap my bioenergy field with the trees' biofield. Then, I used consciously focused energy-healing methodologies with the Birches' internal processes so that their inner functionality would become more efficient.

Another tree, this time near a golf course in West Virginia was in a life-or-death situation. As I walked the perimeter of the golf course in springtime checking the trees, I heard a loud and plaintive cry for help in my inner hearing from behind an adjacent house. The tree had no leaves even though surrounding trees were leafing out abundantly. I went over and put my hands on it.

The tree was in a dilemma. It was concerned about using up its remaining resources to push out leaves from its buds for the new season since it did not think it could make more food to sustain itself once it pushed out those leaves. It knew it had only so much food-resources.

Golf Course Tree: *"If I use that food to push out new leaves, and I can't make more food for myself, then I can't sustain myself. I will die."*

The tree was going to just sit there; it wasn't going to use that energy up to push out new leaves since it didn't think it could make more food for itself.

During the intuitive bioenergy overlap of treatment, I discovered a major disconnect between photosynthesis and circulation. The tree already knew about it. Once I understood the tree's dilemma and used my healing techniques to connect photosynthesis and circulation, the tree said this.

Golf Course Tree: *"I'll push out my leaves now because I know I can make more food for myself and survive."*

I think this shows the deep intelligence within Nature. The tree was aware—on some level—about its dilemma. It didn't know how to get out of it. But, it did know that if it saved its resources by not pushing out leaves, that would give it more time to survive. I simply helped it become more efficient.

For more stories, please see the book: *The Tree Whisperer's 10 Tree and Plant Insights.*

Here are some comments from workshop graduates as they share their experiences and messages.

Carol, gardener: *"My girlfriend likes to hold a party once a year when her enormous Cherry tree blooms. During the celebration, she asked all of us to touch the tree and get a message from it. Most of the people attending had not taken the Tree Whispering class; they reported that the tree was happy and grateful to her for her love. That was probably true; at the same time I got a message that was somewhat disturbing but certainly practical. It said, "I am suffocating and need to breathe." I looked around and saw that my girlfriend's patio was made of bricks that were laid too close to the trunk of the Cherry tree, covering much of the root area. I told her that the tree "said," that it needed* to get air into its roots; it needed to have some of the bricks removed."

Alana, massage therapist: "I was walking around a nature park with my family. A young Maple caught my attention and communicated to me through my intuition, "Snake!" I jumped, but there was no snake there. I didn't understand why the tree would say that to me, but I put my hands on it and said "thank you" to it anyway. As I walked farther along the path, I saw a low stonewall that meandered in and out of the field in a serpentine fashion. I laughed out loud because the tree had been my tour guide."

Leslie, project manager: "Trees talk to me in the rustling of their leaves and movement of their branches, sending messages about themselves and the planet, and in receiving them. I enter into partnership with them."

Georgette, postal worker and homeowner: "A friend gave me a small red Azalea bush, which I planted in my front yard. After a few years, I noticed that it wasn't growing much. So, I talked with it, and it said it was lonely. It wanted a companion. But, it specified that it did not want another red one. It gave me a clear picture of a white Azalea and showed me—in my mind's eye—where nearby to plant the new one. I marked the spot with a stick and left to get the companion. Now, both are growing happily."

Carol, homeowner: "My Japanese Maple is a favorite. When it was young, it looked small and roundish *so I gave it a name: R2-San. Acknowledging the tree with a name is a kind of recognition for it. So, I find that I pay more attention to it. As I was doing the techniques from the Tree Whispering workshop, I heard it say, "I want to grow, to grow tall, and be bigger."*

Here are some messages from the trees and plants themselves:

Plants in an Ornamental Garden in Seattle, Washington State: *"We don't mind too much that the humans cut us back into shapes and sizes. It is like a haircut for us. Overall, the humans are caring to us as best they can from their point of view. However, if the humans would ask us how we should be shaped and cut—if they would come from our point of view—we would be far more beautiful than anything the humans could imagine."*

Maple tree in New York: *"Touch us. Communicate with us. We can share this healing as a cooperative task. We are eager to offer messages to people. We want people to arise as our partners!"*

"To understand is to perceive patterns."
—Isaiah Berlin

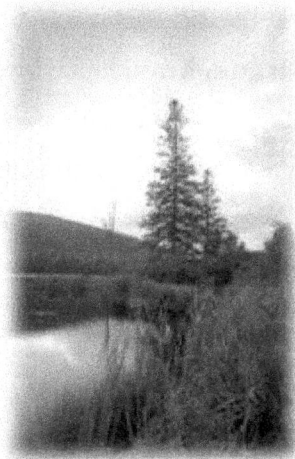

Chapter 5: Meditating On Sacred Trees

Céline Cloutier (Gulabo)

Trees are amongst the oldest beings on this planet and they have always been a very strong influence in people's lives, shares Céline Cloutier (Gulabo) in this section on Sacred Trees.

Tree meditation allows us to consciously connect with the wisdom and natural intelligence of nature. It is easy and enjoyable. Even without speaking of meditation, many people experience well-being just sitting by a tree. I call it the magic of trees!

75

Think back to the last time you truly noticed the shape, color, trunk, branches, flowers, and fruit of a tree? When you did, how did it make you feel?

I know if I spend time with nature, I come back refreshed, rested, lighter, happy and calmer. Since we do not always manage to get outdoors, let's bring the trees to you through the power of meditation!

What are the trees that come forth in your memory and imagination? Which of all the trees you have known, heard, or imagined feels sacred for you? Is it a famous tree, like the Bodhi tree beside which Buddha awakened to enlightenment 2,500 years ago? Is it the Tree of Life found in many traditions, like the Yggdrasill in the Norse tradition of Scandinavia or the sacred Yew in England? Is it the Cedar of Lebanon, whose wood was used to build the first and second temples in Jerusalem?

Each tree has its own particular essence, message, vibration and unique quality which can benefit us. If I ask you to describe an Oak tree, most will say words like "strong" or "grounding." How about the Weeping Willow? Most of us will agree on its flexibility, the sense of water, and the feeling of comfort.

Exercise #1 Your Sacred Tree Meditation

In this meditation we will use visualization and imagination with the purpose of comfort, deep rest and calming the mind. This meditation will last about 15-20 minutes.

Your role is to remain the witness and observe without judgement.

Once you have the feel of this meditation, I invite you to record it as your own personal guided meditation and to listen to it often. Follow your inner call to the place within you of beauty, freedom, joy and love. This is who you really are.

Now it is time for the sacred tree meditation.

You may turn on some quiet music of your choice (optional).

Sit comfortably, feet on the ground and take three deep breaths into the belly.

With each exhalation, locate any tension in the body and with conscious intention, let it go. If more than three breaths are needed, go ahead and take the time you need then continue with the meditation.

Now imagine that you transform yourself and become a magnificent, Sacred Tree. It could be an imaginary tree or one you know.

Vibrational essences from trees support the meditation process. With the Sacred Tree Meditation, I suggest using the Manifestation Essence, because it helps us to direct our imagination, and to perceive and manifest one's truth.

The essences, or specially prepared tinctures, of trees are each linked with certain characteristics like "opening up possibilities" or "enhancing patience."

In the Manifestation Essence are:

1. Bigleaf Maple (*Acer macrophyllum*) *Possibilities*

2. Japanese Walnut (*Juglans ailantifolia*) *Patience, Perseverance*

3. Red Maple (*Acer rubrum*) *Passion, Compassion*

4. Subalpine Fir (*Abies lasiocarpa*) *Peak experience, Transcend limits*

5. White Elm (*Ulmus americana*) *Happiness, Joy*

Take this time to imagine your body rising straight and tall as the solid trunk. See its size, color, and texture. Now, feel you are the tree in its full presence, from the tips of its roots spreading deep and wide into the earth, growing from its trunk into its branches and twigs and expressing itself in its leaves or needles, flowers, and fruit.

Look around, notice where you are. Notice the sky, see the ground and surroundings. Feel and smell the air, listen to sounds, notice all activities, birds, creatures, water, wind...Take a moment right there and breathe.

Now, feel that your legs and feet are extending and merging with the deep and wide roots growing into the earth. Let the roots be strong. Feel that you are firmly grounded into the earth. Take a moment there and breathe. Take some moments here to feel the tree you are!

Imagine an invigorating energy flowing into your entire tree-body from the earth up through the roots...Take a moment and feel this energy travel now into your entire being...Breathe like a tree is breathing, gently, without any effort, soothing...

Enjoy this moment and the sensation of unity with earth and the universe around you.

Continue and imagine this earthy energy purifying each organs, all toxins and blockages. Do not worry, it knows how. Spend a little extra time where ever you feel necessary. Take your time and breathe in all you need.

Now, imagine your arms opening up like branches. Reach as high as you feel, stretch your tree out into the sky. Feel the amazing sensation that it creates in you. Stretch out until you can no longer...

With this new expansion as being a full grown body-tree, go into your heart space and feel the heartbeat...Give thanks for life...Open your heart bigger than ever and let yourself fall into love...Enjoy this moment as your heart fills up with joy, gratitude and grace...Notice what is happening in your entire being right now.

In this peaceful state, imagine coming from above, the warmth of the sun shining onto your tree-body. Let the rays warm up each part of the tree you are...At this time, feel ONE with mother earth...father sky...and being nourished with all the gifts available. Enjoy this moment...Take it all in.

When you feel you have completely taken in the feeling of the tree, where ever you are, you may begin to gradually reconnect with your body feel your feet, your legs, your body, arms, shoulders and head. Breathe a little deeper now and take a nice deep breath.

Come back remembering that you are the tree arising from the earth upon which the sun shines. Know that you are ONE with the pure intelligence of the rhythm of nature. Your breath and your heart are one with Universe.

Two Simple Daily Meditations

In general, meditation in all forms has been known to reduce stress, improve breathing, bring clarity of mind and overall health while nurturing our spirit and allowing us to open to love, beauty and a sense of the sacred.

Meditations are of great benefit when done on a regular basis, and additionally helpful when one is tired, feeling overwhelmed, or when you would simply like to take of break from day to day activities. As we meditate regularly, we gradually remember that we are connected to something beyond, that we are not an island apart from the whole. We remember that there is a place within where all possibilities reside. We remember God or something greater than ourselves.

These two simple meditations, Breath Awareness and Mantra Meditation may be done sitting by a tree.

To experience peace does not mean that your life is always blissful. It means you are capable of tapping into a blissful state of mind amidst the normal chaos of a hectic life.
—Jill Bolte Taylor

Exercise #2 Breath Awareness

The Breathe Essence (Synergy no. 5) helps us connect with our vital force, the subtle energy of our breath. It helps us take life in fully, filter, and let go.

In the Breath Essence are:
1. Apple (*Malus sp.*) *Health, Vigor*
2. Red maple (*Acer rubrum*) *Passion, Compassion*
3. White elm (*Ulmus americana*) *Happiness, Joy*
4. Lilac (*Syringa vulgaris*) * Blessings*

Breath Awareness: Simply take three deep belly breaths.

Take a minute to locate tension in the body. Breathe it out.

Become attentive to your natural breath. Notice the air coming in and out of your nose.

Your only action here is to remain a witness of this activity. Witness your breath and stay with it.

When the mind distracts you, gently come back to your breath.

Sit as long as you have time, 20 minutes, 40 minutes, even an hour. Repeat this meditation as often as you can during your week.

Keys to Mantra Meditation

Take time to sit comfortably, and then take 3 deep belly breaths to release any tension before settling in to chant.

Be a little disciplined. Doing it every day brings many benefits and allows the process to deepen. I recommend 20 minutes each day, but even 10 minutes each day will allow the effects of meditation to accumulate in your life.

Start repeating your Mantra out loud. Continue repeating your mantra, without forcing, without any particular rhythm, changing pitch as it naturally happens. It may follow your breath or not.

At a certain point, you may take the mantra within, either saying it in a soft voice or silently.

If the mind distracts you, as soon as you realize you have been "away," gently come back to repeating your mantra.

Don't mind the mind.

Sit for as long as you have time! Repeat this meditation often.

Here is another tip about the sound of mantras: play with the sounds. *"Ahhh"* seems to correspond to the heart. *"Eee,"* as in the French *"Qui"* or (*"weee"*) corresponds to the crown or top of the head, the connection with the highest self or consciousness.

The sounds in mantras resonate and fill our auric fields. Likewise, tree essences support our energetic well being. The trees in the Universal Essence help us gather healing resources and in restoration. Together these trees seal breaks in our auric field.

In the Universal essence are:

1. Black Cherry (*Prunus erotina*) Cheerfulness*
2. Three Lilacs (*Syringa spp.*) *Open to receive blessings*
3. Mountain Maple (*Acer spicatum*)*Healing matrix*
4. Pacific Yew (*Taxus brevifolia*) *Protection, boundaries*
5. Witch-Hazel (*Hamamelis virginiana*) *Clarity, Vision*

"I keep drawing the trees, the rocks, the river, I'm still learning how to see them; I'm still discovering how to render their forms. I will spend a lifetime doing that. Maybe someday I'll get it right."
—Alan Lee

Exercise #3 Mantra Meditation

A mantra is a word or sound one repeats, for the purpose of meditation.

It can be very effective if you use a word you love.

Masaru Emoto in his books of *Messages from Water* shows images of water crystals that have been exposed to a beautiful word such as *"Thank you."*

Positive words create beautiful water crystal images! If you take a vibrational tree essence or chant a beautiful mantra, you may be changing the water in your body to resonate with what is higher and more harmonious.

A few suggestions about words that you can use as a mantra:

Osho has given the word *"One"* as a mantra. It is powerful. Repeat *"one"* (make the sound long and extended) and feel you are one with your body-mind, the environment, people, animals, and trees, and then expand into the cosmos feeling one with the earth, moon, planets, stars and galaxies. It is a wonderful meditation.

Go and a sit by a tree and chant *"One"* and feel yourself one with the tree. Then you may experience a deep closeness and intimacy with the tree that can be healing and joyful.

Other beautiful words are: *"Thank You,"* *"Love," "Peace,"* and *"Yes."*

Feel the quality of each of these words. Go and chant them by a tree whenever you can and this will amplify the blessing. When you say any of these words, extend the sound, and accent them in a way that fits for you with their meaning.

As French is my mother tongue, says Céline Cloutier (Gulabo), I like the word *"Oui,"* which means *"Yes,"* in the French language. It is pronounced like *"wee"* in English, which children say when they are doing something joyful. Say it with heart and it is a wonderful word that can fill you with a positive resonance.

The specific trees varied between different cultures and geographic locations, but those believed to be "sacred" shared certain traits. Unusual size, beauty, the wide range of materials they provided, unique physical characteristics, or simply the power of the tree's spirit could grant it a central place in the folklore and mythology of a culture.
—Ed Collins, Ravenwoodgrove.org/tree_essays.html

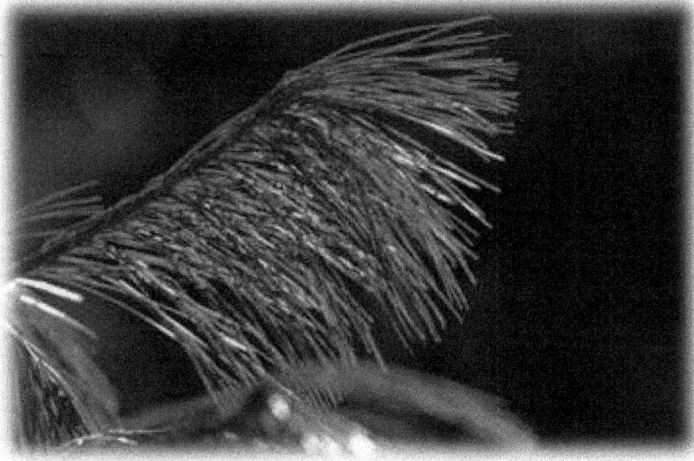

Chapter 6: Learning from Sacred Trees Poems

Kimberly Burnham

There is healing in poetic words and the images they provoke. As you read this book, think of what trees evoke in you and what the words here penned for healing call to mind, says Kimberly Burnham. The images stirred up and painted have healing power. Notice what they bring to you.

Healing Words

Poets create
words strung together
branching and rising
into the air like powerful trees
each leaf carries a message
gentle airy insights
connected in space

Healing words
create vivid images
mind's eye
rising to the challenge
reaching deep
into rich black earth

The body and mind
find a way forward
nourished with
the red heat of a Japanese Maple
poignancy of a Weeping Willow
strengthened
struck with awe by an Oak

Write your own desires
shared like carbon dioxide

on the out breath
with the world's trees

Experience tenderness
newly unfurled bits of green
the beat of water rising to the highest pinnacle
goals achieved
contributions made
to life on earth
grounded in space
adapting through time
connecting the sky and the earth

"Again, and maybe the last time on this earth, I recall the
great vision you sent me. It may be that some little root of
the Sacred Tree still lives. Nourish it then, that it may leaf
and bloom and fill with singing birds. Hear me, not for
myself, but for my people; I am old. Hear me that they may
once more go back into the Sacred Hoop and find the good
red road, the shielding tree."
—Black Elk, from *Black Elk Speaks*

Strong Drives, Health Abounds in Tall Trees

Tall trees branching into deep dark night
waking mornings reaching for what they may
'cause water flows to the tip top light

Struggling to reach and by seedlings do right,
a diverse green, red, yellow, and brown are they
tall trees branching into deep dark night

Rising again blue birds to house in sight
unseen currents lapping at the edge of the bay
'cause water flows to the tip top light

Catching sunbeams spread open like a kite
joy finding space in shade and freedom both okay
tall trees branching into deep dark night

Watching decades pass savoring moments in delight
knowing that now is the time to experience this day
'cause water flows to the tip top light

Health abounds, where is your tip top height
consciousness bending for what you pray
tall trees branching into deep dark night
'cause water flows to tip top light

Tiny Beginnings

One cell grows
a seed, an embryo
experiencing love
wind and water,
storm clouds sunlight
all the diverse experiences
of life
for decades or centuries

Reaching into the earth
drawing out nourishment
creating a home for many
food and love for countless
ones that are similar and different

Then when the towering ones
crash to the earth
with hope and kindness
we leave behind
a lifetime of gifts
gone in body
but generosity and memories forever
for those whose stand now
where we stood

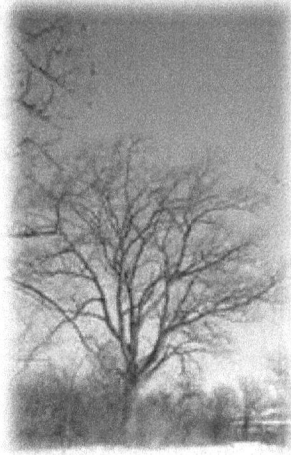

Chapter 7: Minding the Trees, Connection Through Time and Space

Daniel Tigner (Hafiz)

Daniel Tigner takes you through a series of meditations meant to connect you to trees and your own inner strengths. These meditations may help ground you in a stronger sense of time and space in which to heal and live.

If you have a chance to listen to the words with your eyes closed pay attention to the feelings they evoke in you and the vividness of the images. Or try sitting in a natural environment, near a tree or grove of trees as you read these words.

"Our house was up high and in the back there was a decline. Being a kid, the decline seemed like it was very big. It was grassy and there were a couple of huge trees and I would lie on that decline and see through the trees into the sky. While lying there, I would sense that I was abiding in Awareness and I was really no different than the trees. It wasn't an objective experience; it was subjective - because I could feel myself, in a manner of speaking, as being no different than anything around me."
—Ramana, American Mystic, *Memoirs of a Happy Man*

"The more often we see the things around us - even the beautiful and wonderful things - the more they become invisible to us. That is why we often take for granted the beauty of this world: the flowers, the trees, the birds, the clouds - even those we love. Because we see things so often, we see them less and less."
—Joseph B. Wirthlin

Meditation #1 Lifecycle of a Giant Conifer

In the forest a giant Conifer over a thousand years old rises so high that you need to stretch backwards and follow its bole along way up to glimpse its top canopy. Can you imagine the process of its life beginning many centuries ago as a seed and then it pushing out of the ground and standing as a tiny seedling no higher than a flower? In its youth that lasts many human lifetimes it will grow briskly, competing with other trees for the light of the sun.

Can you also see this tree in your mind's eye in old age, one day falling with a great crash to the forest floor where while it decays it will serve as home to many forest creatures? Then finally it disappears, reabsorbed into the earth as vital nutrients that will nourish other plants as they grow.

Our mind is like an amazing time machine that in an instant can transport us across space and time, just as you did a moment ago while imagining the entire life cycle of a tree from seed to old age and beyond. We can use this capacity of our mind to experience again our basic connection with trees.

This in itself is beautiful and healing and will support us in opening to the resonance of the trees. Therefore, as we use our mind in the following sections to explore our connection with trees you may not be surprised to discover how easy it is to recall whatever you have known. Furthermore, these recollections may not occur in a cold and distant way, but feel warm and alive to the point that you are able to recapture the inner core of what made those past experiences important to you. Then mind can move ahead into another time and place, preparing you for deeper possibilities of feeling, sensing and enjoying.

"Trees hold us to our sacred space. They allow us to be all that we can be in that place. This is a wonderful thing. We can feel sacred, secure, and safe.

Ask a child, what do they want to do when they go out and play? "Grandma may I go out and play by the tree?"

They do not ask if they can go out and play in my flower garden. I have a beautiful rose garden. They do not want to play in my rose garden. They say, "Grandma, can I go out and climb the tree? Grandma, can I go out and swing in the tree? Trees connect with children and children love to hug trees. Have you ever hugged a tree? Can you feel the vibration of a tree? It is wonderful."
—Alicia Rocco, Healer and Teacher

Meditation #2 Finding a Beautiful Tree Memory

If you were to remember a time in the past, perhaps recently or perhaps as a child, when you felt deeply connected with a tree, what was that like? You may recall where you were and what you did.

Perhaps you climbed the tree, played around it or enjoyed it in some other way. If your memory is from when you were a child you might recall what it felt like to be in that younger body, how alive you were, and the sensations of the elements like wind and sun or clouds and rain. You might even have felt a certain kind of friendliness with the tree or some other emotion that you may not have paid particular attention to at that time, but which now you can re-experience.

It is beautiful to collect (in the same way that bees collect the nectar from the flowers of trees) the core quality of that past happening. As you do so, you might not be surprised to note that a deeply satisfying feeling remains with you as we move ahead now in our time machine to another time and place.

Meditation #3 Sense of Place in Time

Bringing with you the deeply satisfying nectar from that earlier experience you can now journey ahead to a point in time where you find yourself in a warm season, feeling safe and secure in the forest. You may take a moment to orient yourself, to gain a general sense of what it feels like in this place.

There is the warmth of the sun. You might become aware of the sensations of air and light, the breeze gently caressing your face and waving through your hair and the fresh, clear air streaming around your body. Green, gold, orange, and many earth colors meet your eyes and light dances through the leaves and branches. You might not be surprised then to find yourself feeling incredibly alive, every sense at its peak.

In this pleasurable state of aliveness, arousal and awareness, is it not easy to feel deeply connected to all the life around you, the sky above and the earth below?

There may be awareness of the sounds of the forest: the movement of creatures, the cracking of wood, the rustling of leaves, the musical songs of birds, the sound of running water, the swaying forest canopy, and even of your own breathing. As you notice your breathing, you can feel the wonderful fresh forest air at the tip of your nose and touching your lips then going inside, its fresh vitality nourishing you with the rising and falling of your chest and belly.

Like an animal in the wild you may discover your sense of smell and taste are amplified. You may find yourself registering the rich earthy aromas and flavors of moss, wood, leaves and greenery and many other subtle nuances of scents and tastes.

What's it like to be surrounded by such beautiful and graceful trees, so full of life? Here in this forest you can feel the current of life energy flowing through the whole of your body down through your head, arms, chest, and belly through your thighs, legs, and feet touching the soft earth. You may know you are of the earth. Arising from the earth the whole of your body feels a renewed strength and joy.

Now as you are aware of the trees, you may naturally feel yourself being drawn towards a particular tree, one that is especially beautiful and welcoming, inviting you as a friend.

Your eyes may take in the tree and your ears listen to its musical sounds. You may smell it, move towards it and reach out to touch it, feeling its texture and aliveness. How does it respond to you, how does it feel to you? It might even feel like a part of you.

Meditation #4 Beginning to Come Back to Now

And as you continue to feel this strength and vitality you might even find yourself having warm feelings as your heart reaches out to this tree and the other life forms around you.

Before you come back you may first wish to say goodbye to the tree, to absorb its love and once more share your heart. You may know that you may return whenever you wish to, but for now it is good simply to collect as much as you can of the inner treasures of being in the forest. These feelings of deep relaxation, strength, sensual aliveness, connectedness and heartfulness are yours, so as you come back to where you are in your body in this moment they remain with you.

Come back fully now to where you are, feeling your body, aware of the sights and sounds, tastes and scents, and sensations of being here now.

"Live this moment. Live it intensely, totally, passionately, and then a Miracle happens."
—Osho

Meditation #5 Being Here and Now

As you are here now, you can recognize that through this time machine, your mind, you have not only journeyed into the past and future but also entered a heightened state of sensitivity. Though you have journeyed you can also recognize that you have been here and now all of that time. This is important to understand because in truth all of those inner treasures and feelings of well being are available to you right now. So whenever you are actually physically in the forest or choosing to go on an inner forest journey, in your own way, or by rereading these passages, you are in fact expanding this state of well being, flowing sensual awareness, strength and receptivity. This state can then become a more familiar terrain, taking a fuller place in your daily, moment to moment life.

"It may be that some little root of the Sacred Tree still lives. Nourish it then, that it may leaf and bloom and fill with singing birds. Hear me, not for myself, but for my people; I am old. Hear me that they may once more go back into the Sacred Hoop and find the good red road, the shielding tree."
—Black Elk, *Black Elk Speaks*

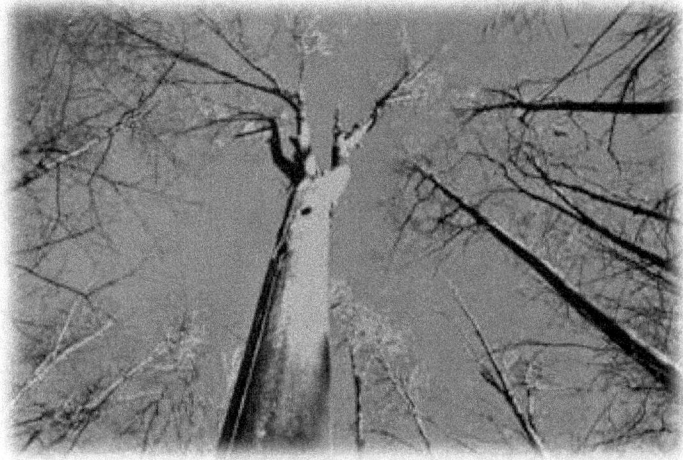

Chapter 8: The Role of Trees

Daniel Tigner (Hafiz)

Trees have evolved within the plant kingdom over the past several hundred million years. These extraordinarily complex biophysical systems transformed the earlier atmospheric conditions on the planet allowing for the evolution of animals and human beings. They are along with other plants the lungs of the planet, releasing daily a fresh supply of oxygen into the atmosphere and storing carbon dioxide through the complex chemical process of photosynthesis in which carbon dioxide, water and the energy of the sun recombine to form oxygen and sugars.

Daniel Tigner (Hafiz) asks you to consider the role of trees in your life and really see the trees around you. How much do you know about historical or famous trees?

Trees hold soil in place protecting streams, hills and farmlands from erosion. They replenish the earth with nutrients, hold water in the ground and help regulate its circulation, act as windbreaks and modify local climates. They serve as homes for insects, birds and animals and as direct food source for both humans and other creatures: pears, apples, bananas, oranges, olives, nuts, spices to name but a few foods.

Trees have an amazing range of uses from wood products, clothing, paper, cork in wine bottles, cinnamon sticks to substances derived from them such as oils, resins and dyes used in making household and industrial products. These include latex for making rubber and other substances utilized in producing cellophane and plastics. The rise and fall of many societies is linked first to the abundance and later decimation of trees and encroaching desertification.

In Mesopotamia, the biblical lands, in Crete and Greece, there were once abundant forests to provide for carpentry, buildings, ships, utensils, fuels and weapons, all those things which human beings use. Those societies grew and flourished until the supply of wood was depleted, then the land was made barren and the soil washed away.

Trees collect energy, heat from the sun, but perhaps other invisible forms of cosmic energy that have been described by, for example, the Chinese and Indians. In China, one name for this energy is chi and in Indian yoga it is called prana. According to yoga, when we breathe we not only take in oxygen, but life energy, as if oxygen is the outer content, and the inner juice is prana. You can call it factor x. Ask why you feel so nourished in the presence of a great tree or in the forest, is it the oxygen alone or the addition of an unbeknown energy factor at work?

A view of North America as it existed in 1600 would show two thirds of the continent covered with vast primordial forests of immense trees. This canopy has been greatly diminished by the 1850's, but there were still large areas of original woods. The acceleration of European immigration brought devastation to the forests as huge tracts of trees were cleared. Not only was there a need for wood, but it is said that trees were seen as a nuisance that had to be cleared away for farms and the growth of the cities. The result was not only a disaster that left only a tiny remnant of the original forest but contributed to the loss of huge amounts of rich soil.

As we grow in understanding of the interdependence of life we begin to reexamine the idea that the earth's treasures are ours to plunder as we wish and take steps to preserve what remains of the original forest for its biodiversity and intrinsic beauty. Without trees it would be a dry and desolate world. Beyond their use by humans and other creatures, trees are beings to be honored in and of themselves.

Perhaps the greatest gift of trees is simply their beauty, the amazing range of colors and forms that please and nourish the eyes. It is no wonder that trees have been worshipped and their presence forms a central motif in history, myths and legends, an example being the tree said to have yielded fruit giving everlasting life in the Garden of Eden known as the Tree of Life. In making healing essences from trees, I have experienced a feeling of urgency, a sense that the trees really want to be heard and seen.

"If we surrendered to earth's intelligence we could rise up rooted, like trees."
—Rainer Maria Rilke, *Rilke's Book of Hours: Love Poems to God*

Trees as Markers of History, Rituals and Spiritual Events

Many of the key events in history are marked by an association with a tree. The enlightenment of Buddha happened under the Bodhi Tree. God speaks to Moses from a Burning Bush. It is a branch from an Olive Tree brought back to Noah's Ark that symbolizes peace, and the document that is a precursor to our modern declarations of human rights, the Magna Carta, is said to have been signed under a tree. The tree on the Connecticut quarter is the 800 year old Charter Oak tree. These are just a few of thousands of examples of trees associated with important events.

Visitors to Canada's capital of Ottawa may see trees planted by dignitaries at the Governor General's estate. People like John F. Kennedy and Jacqueline Kennedy both planted Red Oaks.

Trees can be important personal markers. We plant trees as memorials for people we have loved.

For many people, one of the most striking symbols of a tree as a marker is, of course, the Christmas Tree.

Christmas is, as are many of our rituals, a time for Christian families and friends to rest, and reflect on our lives, and often a time for healing.

The rest of us can look at the connection to trees and light and consider our own connection to something greater than ourselves.

We can each ponder the impact of trees in our lives and the impact of our lives on others.

"Rituals and myths, such as those involving Christmas and Santa Claus, are among the few remaining links to our ancient roots; they are part of the most tenacious and most important myth of all — the story of man's first awareness of being part of something greater than himself and of the shattering memory of the conquest of fire; that fiery instant which totally changed the fate of mankind."

—Tony van Renterghem, from the fascinating and highly original book: *When Santa was a Shaman — The Ancient Origins of Santa Claus & the Christmas Tree*

O Christmas Tree ("O Tannebaum")

O Christmas Tree, O Christmas Tree,
Your branches green delight us.
They're green when summer days are bright;
They're green when winter snow is white.
O, Christmas Tree, O Christmas Tree,
Your branches green delight us!

O Christmas Tree, O Christmas Tree,
You give us so much pleasure!
How oft at Christmas tide the sight,
O green fir tree, gives us delight!
O Christmas Tree, O Christmas Tree,
You give us so much pleasure!

Oh Christmas Tree, Oh Christmas Tree
Forever true your colour.
Your boughs so green in summertime
Stay bravely green in wintertime.
Oh Christmas tree, Oh Christmas tree
Forever true your colour.

Oh Christmas tree, Oh Christmas tree
You fill my heart with music.
Reminding me on Christmas Day
To think of you and then be gay.

Oh Christmas tree, Oh Christmas tree
You fill my heart with music.

O Christmas tree, O Christmas tree!
How are thy leaves so verdant!
Not only in the summertime,
But even in winter is thy prime.
O Christmas tree, O Christmas tree,
How are thy leaves so verdant!

O Christmas tree, O Christmas tree,
Much pleasure dost thou bring me!
For every year the Christmas tree,
Brings to us all both joy and glee.
O Christmas tree, O Christmas tree,
Much pleasure dost thou bring me!

O Christmas tree, O Christmas tree,
Thy candles shine out brightly!
Each bough doth hold its tiny light,
That makes each toy to sparkle bright.
O Christmas tree, O Christmas tree,
Thy candles shine out brightly!

Ode to Connecticut's Charter Oak

Kimberly Burnham

Already 500 years old
in 1662 Governor John Winthrop Jr.
wins a charter
the right to exist here
in the forests of Connecticut
okay from a far says King Charles II
he does not see this October day flush
with reds and yellows

A nation state early in birth throws
witnessed by a old Oak tree
a Charter on paper
earlier grown in a European forest
a human generation passes
the 500 year old Oak sees
the minions of James II ride
to take the Charter back

Suddenly the room darkens
light returns with candle bright
the charter gone from the table
hidden in a 13th century white oak tree

commemorated on Connecticut's quarter

An object of veneration
by generations of native Americans
traditionally holding their councils
beneath its expanses

Not until 1614 did the old tree
became the property of Samuel Wyllys,
an early Hartford landowner
busy clearing away the homestead forest
circling ever closer to the white oak
visited he was by a delegation of native Americans
fearful that their revered tree
destroyed would be
pleading for the Oak
planted as a token of peace
by a great Sachem

The appearance of springtime leaves
communication from the Great Spirit
begin again

And so the ancient tree stood
until a great storm on August 21, 1856
civic mourning ensued
the day the Charter Oak fell

an honor guard placed
around the remains
attaching an American flag
to the shattered trunk
Colt's Band of Hartford
a funeral dirge played
at sunset Hartford bells
rang out

From near and far
people gathered
even the smallest fragments
of the oak passed along to posterity
precious reminders of heritage
and freedom

Acorns dropped by the great tree
gathered and planted
producing in time
a forest of trees
descended from the historic oak

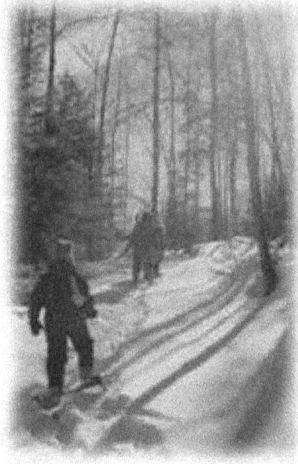

Chapter 9: Environmentalists and Faith Leaders Join Hands

Kimberly Burnham

When did you last hug a tree? How do you feel when you stand in stillness in a grove of tree and listen? Listening to the sound of the wind, the beating of your own heart, or your intuitive sense. What do you hear?

Groves of trees can be beneficial in many ways. We can access the divine in a different way from worship in temples or manmade structures. We can enjoy the beauty and utility of biodiversity. We can eliminate some of the carbon footprint created by our lives.

In the *"Trees, Forests, and the Sacred"* session at the 2015 Parliament of Religions, Jason Minton Brown, explained how environmentalists, naturalists, and people concerned with biodiversity and deforestation are reaching out to religious groups for help in preserving sacred groves. Together they are saving and maintaining thousands of sacred trees and natural sites.

The LDS (Mormon) church helps maintain and preserve four sacred groves or natural areas. One grove is known as the Sacred Grove where Joseph Smith had his first revelatory experience in Palmyra, New York; also in New York the Hill Cumorah; Joseph Smith's birth place in Vermont; and another revelation site in Pennsylvania are all maintained by the LDS church. Noting that the LDS church bought the Palmyra site in the 1920's, Brown said, Robert Parrott, a forester and naturalist employed by the Church, is working to bring the Sacred Grove back to its natural state or the way it was in late 1820's.

In a 2012 tree metaphor entitled, *"Stand in the Sacred Grove,"* Elder Marlin K. Jensen of the LDS church noted several life lessons from the Sacred Grove.

1. Trees always grow toward the light.

2. Trees require opposition to fulfill the measure of their creation.

3. Trees are best grown in forests, not in isolation.

4. Trees draw strength from the nutrients created by previous generations of trees.

Describing some of the many sacred groves or forests around the world, Brown explained how in Estonia, one of the places in Europe with the least organized religion, a majority of people believe trees have souls. They have 550 preserved groves and 2000 Hiis (Estonian for sacred trees).

Brown's PhD research is on the perceptions and management of Catholic monastic landscapes in the American West. While his religious roots are in the LDS (Mormon) Church, he has recently begun practicing Zen Buddhism and Catholicism. He is a founding member of the Salish Sea Spiritual Ecology Alliance, a civil society organization dedicated to Inter-path ecology work.

He talks about how in Thailand, where logging is destroying huge tracts of land, monks have started ordaining tree and wrapping them in robes in order to protect them. In some cases logger don't cut the trees because they know they are sacred. To what lengths would you go to preserve the trees on your

114

land or in your community? To what lengths would you go to preserve your quality of life and the air you breathe?

In Haiti, where deforestation is having disastrous consequences, the Mapou tree, considered sacred is not being cut down. There is a similar story with a Great Oak in Northern California which is thought to be 2000 year old and the Mahabodhi tree (ficus) in Bodh Gaya, India. There are nearly 150,000 sacred tree sites or forests throughout India, which are being preserved because of naturalists and people of different faith traditions are working together.

In Fish Lake, not far from Salt Lake City, where the Parliament of Religions was held there is a quaking aspen grove that is possibly the largest organism in the world. The root system covers 100 acres and it could be 300,000 years old, said Brown.

What trees are "sacred" in your community or to you?

Thus were the visions of mine head in my bed:
I saw, and behold
A tree in the midst of the earth,
and the height thereof was great.
The tree grew, and was strong,
and the height thereof reached
Unto heaven, and the sight thereof

115

to the end of all the earth.
—King James Version, Daniel 4:10-11

"Her eye fell everywhere on lawns and plantations of the freshest green; and the trees, though not fully clothed, were in that delightful state when farther beauty is known to be at hand, and when, while much is actually given to the sight, more yet remains for the imagination."
—Jane Austen

"The birth and death of leaves is part of that greater cycle that moves among the stars."
—Rabindranath Tagore, poet, Nobel Laureate

"The forest is the source of everything in the world, the dharma, the natural law. It is the university of our life and understanding, the place where Buddha first had a revelation, where monks first came into existence."
—Prajak Kuttajitto, Thailand.

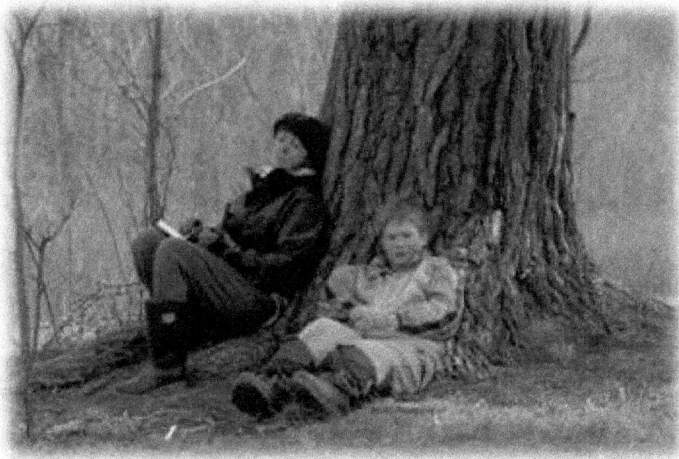

Chapter 10: Awakening, Trees, and Your True Self

Céline Cloutier (Gulabo)

In this section, Céline Cloutier (Gulabo) answers questions like, what is vibration and how does understanding trees help us with self-actualization? She wants to share about seven amazing trees that assisted me tremendously before, during and after this passage. This is the story of finding joy with self-awareness, consciousness and a set of seven special trees. These trees came together in an essence we created called WOVE short for Women's Own Vibrational Essence.

"Happiness held is the seed; Happiness shared is the flower."
—John Harrigan

"Actions are the seed of fate deeds grow into destiny."
—Harry S Truman

"We cannot conceive of matter being formed of nothing, since things require a seed to start from... Therefore there is not anything which returns to nothing, but all things return dissolved into their elements."
—William Shakespeare

Everything is Vibration

Have you heard this expression: *"Everything is vibration?"* What does it really mean?

Quantum physics reveals that everything including ourselves and all things in the environment are created of microscopic vibrational chords found in the center of infinitesimally small atoms. Invisible to the naked eye, their effects are active and can be measured.

Everything is vibrational!

If all is vibration, you may contemplate these questions:

Are we then all connected?
Do we vibrate together as one?
Why do I sometimes or always feel alone, separated?
What is total freedom?
What is my purpose in life?
What is Enlightenment? Is that possible?
What are your beliefs concerning success, love, health?

"It is remarkable how closely the history of the apple tree is connected with that of man."
—Henry David Thoreau

Your Birthright

"You are wholeness, you are pure love, you deserve it all, and that is your birthright!" If I say this to you, how does that make you feel? Why?

Take a moment to reflect, breathe, observe, breathe some more, and observe what comes up! No judgement, just watch and see what happens.

Self Realization

Now, a true story!

On July 4th 1999, unconditional love, unity consciousness, divine light or call it what you like, crept up on and in me unexpectedly and gracefully. This emerging happened to occur after several years of meditation and a knowing that I was connected to the pure intelligence of the rhythm of nature. This transformation translated into an ongoing, moment-to-moment realization.

In a Guided Meditation introduced by Oprah Winfrey, Dr. Deepak Chopra said: *"Your TRUE SELF is closer than your breath."* It is. And yes, *"It"* can reveal itself at any moment - because it is who we are, and our nature. We have just forgotten it, just as we forget to breathe sometimes, or we forget that behind dark clouds, the sun remains there.

This is it! This moment is the simple realization of non-duality that we are born whole, and it is up to us to believe it. It is as certain as knowing that the sun rises in the morning. No matter what, I know "*It*" now and I know that you somewhere, know it too!

Living in the Light

When I am asked to describe what *"Living in the Light is,"* I find myself using words such as bliss, happiness, joy, and freedom from unfounded worries. There is faith, trust, abundance, unconditional love.....

And how does it manifest itself in my life? I always see that desires are fulfilled before they become desires!

So now, before I go on about that particular day, July 4ᵗʰ 1999:

Take a moment and ask yourself, "*who am I?*" For example, "*I am a woman.*"

Go within, and after each answer, ask again, "*Who am I?*" Ask until there is NO more answer. In that space, breathe, observe without judgement, wait, observe, and if something comes up, listen, breathe, observe and feel what happens.

Take a moment and ask yourself, what is living in the light? For example *JOY*.

List everything and take a moment to observe how each item on your list makes you feel. Breathe, and observe without judgement.

Satori: an Experience of Delight

"There is one unity, unified wholeness, total natural law, in the transcendental unified consciousness."
—Maharishi Mahesh Yogi

I remember in 1985 when I first started studying Transcendental Meditation (TM), I was 24 years old and TM provided a wonderful structure and foundation to connect with inner peace. I understood that a teacher living in India wearing a white robe and with a white beard was behind this work. That was Maharishi Mahesh Yogi. The word "Enlightenment" was mentioned often, but with French as my first language, I did not know what it meant. Even when I sort of understood the word, it felt like it was not my concern - I simply enjoyed my practice daily.

I used to listen to Maharishi during retreat weekends. I could not understand a word as he spoke because of his accent and the words being so foreign. I just enjoyed his smile and lovely cheeks and I was attracted to this energy. I just sat and enjoyed the vibration!

Hafiz (aka Daniel Tigner, I call him by his spiritual name of Hafiz, given by Osho. I also have a spiritual name from Osho, Ma Sunder Gulabo), my partner in *Canadian Forest Tree Essences*, had graciously invited me to meet an "Enlightened Being" for my birthday. Francis Lucille was coming to a center nearby to give a retreat and holding a Satsang meditation that was open to visitors. I thought, *"Oh, here is this word "Enlightenment" again."*

My first reaction as I sat on the floor in front of this gentle man was, *"Oh, what is the fuss, this man has nothing I do not have!"* I listened to his answers as people proceeded with questions. The words did not matter so much, but the feeling of calm, and peace was embracing the room and me.

One day after that, Francis called me at home. He was coming back into the area and he wanted to invite my son to ski with him and his son, as the two boys were close in age. During our conversation, something extraordinary happened. As we were simply exchanging about very ordinary stuff concerning my son's visiting with his son for the trip skiing, we somehow got into a conversation about whether he should bring his bathing suit. We became silly and ended up speaking about polka dot bikinis!!

We were into an amazing flow of energy.....and, at that moment, I suddenly experienced what is called a Satori - a moment of total bliss. We laughed at nothing and everything. It was awesome in the truest sense! Then we hung up.

Ask Your True Self

I invite you to see how you can express living in the light in your life? Taking my example of Joy, it might be as simple as, *"I could eat an ice cream cone more often! That brings me joy."*

Take a moment and ask yourself, what is my purpose in life? What do I wish to experience? For example love!

Take a moment and ask yourself, what do I wish to learn in life for growth? For example, to meditate!

Take a moment and ask yourself what contribution do I wish to make in this life? For example, write a book?

For each question look at the physical, emotional, intellectual and spiritual levels. Once you have your list for each section, take one or two items of your choice and do the following:

Ask yourself - using my example of Experiencing Love, Learning How to Meditate, Contributing by Writing a Book; if these were already accomplished, how would it make me feel?

Then Vibrate with it! See it! Breathe it! Rejoice! Celebrate!

And finally, let it go!

Reborn on the 4th of July

"...start with the idea, with this climate around you, with this vision: Let it be declared to your every cell of your body and every thought of your mind, let it be declared to every nook and corner of your existence, that: "I am a Buddha."
—Osho

I had been involved with the tree essences project for a year or so. I had also started one year of Osho active meditations to help cleanse emotions and old stuff!

125

About OSHO: I now understand that Osho—that indescribable mystic—came into my life at a time when another level of consciousness was necessary to continue to evolve. I remember the first time I listened to a video of him speaking. He made me smile. I was never very attentive to the words he said, but to the entire energy and vibration around him. His presence was a guiding energy on that day of transformation, July 4, 1999.

Early on that July 4th, I was not feeling my best. My body was aching and strong feelings were arising. I was guided by Hafiz, who was feeling attuned to and guided in the words he spoke to me by Osho, to go inward and just feel, observe, stay with whatever was coming up, remaining still, not judging, and witnessing. After a few moments of this exercise and by the grace of love, a moment of swirling occurred where I almost got scared of losing control. But again, I was guided to not do anything and what was meant to happen, happened.

It was like the entire universe entered this body and created a stirring motion within to flush all the nonsense out of me. I kept watching while this was happening, while tears started running gently. I was simply a witness to this procession - in awe - until all of a sudden; it just stopped and left the premises.

At that moment, I got it! There was nothingness, emptiness filled with joy, peace, love, space. I got it! And I knew that it was there all the time. I saw that I had been living with fear, anger, and all the silly make-believe emotions for nothing. I got that this state of being is the only truth!

The Unbearable Lightness of Being

Then what happened?

I opened my eyes filled with tears of relief and deep rest. I felt so much space within and without. It seemed like this body was too small to contain this much. It seemed like the only thing I could do was to take one step and then another. I was floating. Can you imagine unloading a life time of garbage off your shoulders. The unbearable lightness of being - that was the experience.

Seven Amazing Trees in Wove

I want to share about seven amazing trees that assisted me tremendously before, during and after this experience. These trees came together in an essence we created called WOVE short for Women's Own Vibrational Essence.

This essence is about juggling with all aspect of a woman's life, celebrating womanhood, and coming together to the center of Who We Are!

The seven trees formed a matrix of energy that in a mysterious and gentle way supported the awakening and transformative process that I underwent!

Blue Beech (Carpinus caroliana),
Eastern White Pine (Pinus strobus),
Euonymus (Euonymus bungeans),
Mock Orange (Philadelphus sp.),
Silver Maple (Acer saccharinum),
Sphagnum Moss (Sphagnum sp.) and
White Birch (Betula papyrifera)

A Grove of Eastern White Cedars

Floating—It seemed like the only sensible thing to do was to go to the trees! These ancient beings knew best. As I lay down in a forest of Cedars, I felt supported and mostly I felt more grounded and understood. They helped me get gradually accustomed to this new state.

Grounding

Every day for a long time I needed to make an effort to ground myself as I could have stayed with my eyes closed, meditating and merging, vibrating, with all there is.

It would have been easy to move to India or some other place and just sit still, but I had a wonderful son at home, a family, friends, a business, a wonderful partner, and many projects still to accomplish. I was wisely guided, and gradually the body got used to this new state and allowing me to experience day-to-day life within this wholeness. I felt blessed and grateful. And the grounding presence of trees made all the difference!

Sharing

Why share this story of my own awakening? Because, this ongoing knowing my True Self as a lived experience, allows me to share a simple and wonderful truth: "Enlightenment" is available to all, to you, since it is you!

A few years after this awakening, when that state had settled in me, we had the privilege of having an awakened teacher, A. Ramana, and a companion,

Elizabeth, stay with us in our home. They had come from North Carolina in the USA for Ramana to give a weekend seminar introducing a process called Self-Inquiry.

When Ramana met me, he gently said: *"Gulabo, you are like a breath of fresh air."* I smiled. One day, Ramana left for a drive with our friend, Saroja, who had organized Ramana's seminar, while Elizabeth stayed with me.

Elizabeth needed to make some follow-up calls. Meanwhile, I was preparing dinner and between calls we spoke. As I was cutting carrots, we shared about the experience of Enlightenment, since this was my knowing by now and Elizabeth had observed Ramana for 30 years ...At one point, I asked Elizabeth, "*And how about yourself?*"

Something happened at the instant of that question. Elizabeth did not say much, but simply smiled. A few weeks afterwards, she sent me a tape telling me about her own awakening in the kitchen that had followed my question. She had simply realised she was there. When she shared with Ramana, his response was: "*It's about time!*"

Love

Awakening can happen at any moment. For me, on that July 4th, it unfolded while we were sitting in a booth in a restaurant I went often to with Hafiz. For Elizabeth, it happened in a simple kitchen, in the midst of cutting vegetables and sharing as friends do. In the bigger course of life, I had known since I was a small child that there had to be something else out there. There was a thirst for more, for love, for knowledge, and yet, I did not know how to find it. Little did I know that the something was not out there, but inside of myself. I was blessed because I had no expectation or demand that something happen: Hafiz always noted that although I was thirsty, I had no direct desire for "Enlightenment" or some kind of attainment. It was by this grace that I was able to remain open and allow everything needed to unfold.

"Now I live a wonderful life, and I have a passion to share light and love with all open to receive. Yet, I also know that nobody can give it to you. Still, you can do all you can to become conscious, open your heart, be a witness of your life so you get to know yourself. Gradually, the imposter you have become will leave the premises - because

it is your birth right to know Your True Self and you deserve all life has in store for you, meaning all."
—Namasté, Ma Sunder Gulabo aka Celine Cloutier

"That's the way I do things when I want to celebrate, I always plant a tree. And so I got an indigenous tree, called Nandi flame, it has this beautiful red flowers. When it is in flower it is like it is in flame."
—Wangari Maathai

"This feeling of being lonely and very temporary visitors in the universe is in flat contradiction to everything known about man (and all other living organisms) in the sciences. We do not "come into" this world; we come out of it, as leaves from a tree. As the ocean "waves," the universe "peoples." Every individual is an expression of the whole realm of nature, a unique action of the total universe. This fact is rarely, if ever, experienced by most individuals. Even those who know it to be true in theory do not sense or feel it, but continue to be aware of themselves as isolated "egos" inside bags of skin."
—Alan Watts, *The Book: On the Taboo, Against Knowing Who You Are*

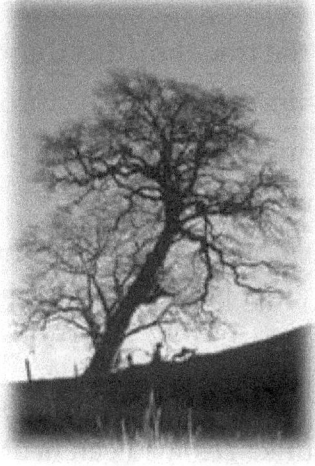

Chapter 11: Seasons of a Tree and a Life

Margo Royce

Have you made a difference in the life of a child? Has a child made a difference in yours? What you learn together will stay with both of you forever.

Listen

Listen, encourages Margo Royce, and consider how listening can help you heal.

Shhh...

Listen to the trees breathe. Can you hear it?
No, not the rustle of the breeze through the leaves.
But that is like music isn't it?

Something deeper...

Yes, that's close. That is the sap running through the tree like its life's blood. The sound of the tree's heartbeat.

Listen closer. Rest your cheek against the bark of this sturdy trunk. Yes, you can hear it now! It is the tree breathing...each breath drawing in carbon dioxide and exhaling beautiful oxygen for us to breathe!

Each breathe healing us and the land.
...The more trees - the more pure the air.

Isn't that amazing! The breath of the trees make it better air for all of us to breathe! What a wonder of nature.

My little girl listened while resting her cheek against the trunk. She wrapped her little arms around the tree. We both gave it a big hug.

Smiling and holding hands, we continued walking through the woods.

"You know," I said in wonder, looking all around, *"every tree is beautiful. I've never seen a tree that wasn't beautiful. And yet, each one is different."*

"Just like people," said my little one.

"Yes, my Darlin', just like people.
Every one different and every one beautiful."

A Kitten's Claws

I'm sure you have heard trees sing and cry. Have you ever heard one laugh? Go tickle one and listen. Squirrels and birds do it all the time.
Sometimes, so do kittens.

Our beautiful black and orange Persian cat, Mika, chased a squirrel up a tree. Mika's instincts were intact but, alas, her claws were not. Bewildered, she slid back down. The tree shook with laughter. Or maybe it was the squirrel.

My daughter, Shanty, wrote in a grade 2 school essay, *"Mika can't have baby kittens because she doesn't have claws."* And the tree shook with laughter again. Or maybe it was her Mom.

A Time to Nest and a Time to Fly

Have you ever pondered whether you are in a safe place or stuck in the mud? Whether you are free to go or needing to be free? You may want to take a week or month to identify which is right for you. This inner conversation

135

may take some time or help from someone caring and knowledgeable. But if you are in a dangerous place, it is time to seek immediate help. It is time to find your wings and fly.

Farewell letter to Erin:
To borrow from Ecclesiastes 3:1
To everything there is a season,
A time for every purpose under heaven…

A time to go and a time to return
A time to fly and a time to nest
A time to seek and a time to find
A time to walk into the unknown
Open to whatever adventures await
And a time to return to the known
With the knowledge you will always have a place there.

This is a season for you to fly and to discover and to witness.
Who knows what sights you will see, what people you will meet,
What challenges you will surmount.
But always know that if you are not happy
You can always come back
For life is for living and enjoying

And if you do not enjoy the experience, you need not
remain in it.

I will miss you of course
I love you and I like you
I'm proud of you and I believe in you
And whether you are in the next room
Or half a world away –
These truths remain constant.

May the people you meet be kind and interesting
The places seen be all worthy of photos
And the experiences that await you be
Wonderful memories in the making.

I'll be on your shoulder when you want it,
And a phone call away when you need it.
Take great good care
And have a magnificent adventure!

     I took Erin to the airport at 5:20 this morning.
She took my envelope with her to read on the plane.
She is on her way to work on an Alaska Cruise Ship.
     At 9:00 a.m. I'm back home and notice the little
female robin making a nest in the tree in front of my
kitchen solarium windows. The kitchen is on the forth
level of my townhouse and puts me at eye level to

this beautiful maple tree and all its visitors. I've been watching her progress all day and it is fascinating. Now, going on 6:00 p.m., she is still at it, having taken no breaks at all.

She brings a mouthful of black and wet material and deposits it between the limbs of the tree. She has built it up considerably all ready by the time I noticed it this morning. She may have started at dawn.

Then, as it gains in material, she drops her mouthful in the centre and distributes it with her beak. As its construction grows, she sits in the middle and builds up the sides with her beak and body, pressing her rosy chest into the sides and up – fluttering her wings and tail to further distribute, then her beak to apply specifics.

It is fascinating. I've never seen the step-by-step process of nest construction close up before. I've never known that the curved bowl of a nest was created by the action of pressing her chest into the sides after flattening the bottom with her body and beak.

By evening, her wee, rosy chest is now dirty from pressing it into the muck from the materials she gathers for 16 cm of snow fell yesterday and all is cold and wet. She is still at it! I watch her throughout the hours and marvel at what a busy little female she is.

Fly – bring back material – distribute – press – move it around – press firmly down and up – fly off. Moments later she will return and repeat. Her mate stays nearby. *"What do you do,"* I wondered. *"Are you guarding? Making sure no other birds steal the material or the nest itself?"*

And there she is—building the nest, laying the eggs, keeping them warm, feeding the babies. I saw that process a few years ago here and was amazed at the constant flying to get food and back to baby over and over all day for hours on end.

And what does he do in this partnership? Not being anti-male but genuinely wondering what besides sperm does he contribute? Well, she's making wonderful progress and given me joy to witness this. I hope she can rest soon. I hope her mate will provide dinner and give her busy little wings a massage tonight! I wonder how she knows what to do and how to do it. How fascinating!

I love my trees, plants, birds and creatures and the miracle of spring bringing all to life right before my eyes. As I wrote to Erin, there is indeed, in all our lives, a time to fly and a time to nest.

As I fall asleep this night, my thoughts are with two busy little females, Erin and the robin. One on the fly, one on the nest.

I take such a wonderful joy in the canopy of the tree in the world beyond my kitchen windows and the creatures who visit.

Within the next two weeks, I try to understand what happens. I wonder if it is something like this: There is a mating. Then, once she feels a stirring, she quickly builds her nest from dawn to dusk in the steps I've described. For a couple of days, she and her mate stayed around but she wasn't in her nest a lot. She seemed to be eating and getting exercise before retiring to her nest. After a couple of days, I believe her eggs had been laid. She would go off briefly for a worm and return. Her mate was no longer around.

On one of her return trips, she stopped on the fence and looked upward to see what was the clatter above her. I had been drawn to the window when loud calls of what I call rooks, dive-bombed a huge crow onto a nearby roof. They kept dive bombing the huge crow while the little robin cocked her head up curiously to watch. The rooks, which I now know to be grackles, chased the crow away, they in hot pursuit. The little robin watched with interest and then returned to her nest.

The following day, I heard more ferocious calls and was amazed to see, with horror, the big crow land in the tree. As the grackles came from all directions, the crow stepped right to the edge of the nest. Next, the little robin returns and she calls out in her own urgent voice as she dive-bombs the crow too! Twice, calling out along with the grackles, she joins them and all swoop and call and dive and the tree is alive with activity and noise as I join in at the kitchen window, clapping loudly and calling out with every bit as much concern as the birds. The crow flies off, the others still in hot pursuit. The little robin returns and seems to stand and count her eggs and make sure they are ok. They seem to be. She settles on top of them and all is quiet in the tree before my kitchen window. She is a brave little soul.

That evening, a high wind swings the boughs of the tree back and forth. I see her feathers ruffled and know the wind to be cold as well as strong. Because the leaves are slow to open this spring, I am able to see clearly but worry that she has so little protection from predators and weather.

A couple of days later, it pours rain and I see her with her wings draped over the nest rather than tucked inside and realize she is keeping the nest dry as well as the eggs...at her expense.

What a lot she has to contend with. What spirit and instinct this little creature displays. What stress she is under! And now, two weeks since she built her nest, the drama in the tree continues and, as it pours

141

rain and the temperature dips down to 2 degrees, I worry for she is soaking wet.

The crow has been back twice more. Thank heavens for the rooks/grackles that protect the little robin's nest while protecting their own. This morning the crow, too, is sodden. I'm afraid for the robin's survival since this heavy, cold rain has not let up since yesterday.

I call the Wild Bird Sanctuary and am told that, yes, she is at risk. They have been receiving calls about purple martins that are so wet they are grounded and can't get back to their nests and eggs. How awful!

If she can just make it through today and tonight, it is to be dry and 14 degrees tomorrow. But still, all this day, weather reports call for more cold, rain and snow to continue overnight with temperatures dropping to zero. I want to climb up and place an umbrella over her nest, to do most anything to protect her and to keep her dry and warm. But I know I can't. My attempt might put her and her eggs at even greater risk. As I look out to her nest before going to bed, I wonder at what a brave, determined little soul she is. I am so afraid her wet little body will freeze. *"Hold on little robin,"* I whisper. *"Hold on until morning."*

This morning I awaken to sunshine and am glad for the robin. When I come downstairs, though, she is not in her nest. I watch and wait. After an hour, I still continue to watch for her but I know she is not coming back. Either she didn't make it through the night or her eggs didn't. Most likely the crow came back in early morning and got the eggs and she has left her nest for good. I feel so sad. She worked so hard for over two weeks and, now, all for naught.

As I watch and worry for the little robin through my kitchen windows, I know I am being silly, casting glances at her nest, still hopeful for her return. I realize the degree of sadness I feel for her is out of proportion to the reality of nature unfolding before me as it does with weather and creatures in all their dramas. She is not my bird but the bird, living in the tree before my window. I admonish myself.

But then I remember her curiosity, tilting her head over and watching something with interest; her courage to defend her unborn babies and attack a huge crow five times her size; her knowledge of how to press her little chest into these scraps and fragments to achieve the perfect shaped nest for herself and her eggs; her valiant behaviour in sheltering both her nest and her eggs from the cold, heavy rain. Knowing that, in spite of a small brain within a small body, there is intelligence, instinct, curiosity, personality and emotion dwelling there.

As I continued to gaze out my window, her mate came round the corner and glanced up at the nest. Almost as if he "knew" automatically, he flew past the side of the house to the big lawn in front. Suddenly understanding, I flew upstairs to my bedroom balcony. There they were, together, nudging each other briefly and she nimbly scooping up all the fat worms drawn to the wet surface. She was agile and active with her mate, nearby, doing the same.

She had gone to the opposite side of the house. She hadn't died in the wet night nor had she left the area for good. Just her nest and just for now. I watched them a long time. Watched her hear something overhead, stop, cock her head and watch with interest the sounds above.

"Oh little robin," I whispered, *"I'm so glad you are ok and together and here."* She seemed to look right up at me. Strangely, she, followed by her mate, flew onto the brick wall on my yard and the two of them stared right up at my balcony. Although it is impossible, it seemed as though the force of my thoughts were so strong, that they picked up on them. Looking up, cocking their heads, they seem to say, *"See, we're ok."*

I realize I am witness to the trees, creatures, birds, plants, weather. I can't make them well or protect them or change danger to safety for them. I can only witness – watch, wonder and learn in the privilege of shared moments.

The little robin worked hard, fought bravely and valiantly but moved on from needing to tend her eggs to living fully in the next moment as well. I have learned they may have three broods this season so I guess they will just wait until the next stirring and do it all again when the time comes. In the meantime, she is healthy and happy and able to eat for herself and gain strength and health and a little rest and relaxation from her busy life as a female robin.

Sometimes, you can't help. You can't save or protect or direct. You can only witness and honour. Witness those you love who will fly or nest as others have had to watch you and I do the same and could not, and should not, have tried to do it for us. A time to trust instincts – those of others, and our own as well. So too for everyone…all creatures great and small.

Fly!!!

Do you consider the differences between taking a risk and the expected results before taking an action? Or do you let the five year old child within take the leap and think about it later? Do you think there is a healthy balance between the two paths to decision making?

You grab hold of the long branch of the tree that grows by the river. You run, you grab and into the river you fly! Unless you are a girl. Girls aren't allowed to do it. That's what my big brother told me. But not if you are alone. Then you fly! Trees won't tell!

Brother and Friend

Have you ever engaged in time travel? You can, you know. You can go back in your memories and re-experience the beautiful people and moments of your life. Can you close your eyes and feel, smell, hear a voice, touch a moment and never let it go? Yes, you can.

My brother, Dale, and I explore the Petrified Forest and Painted Desert the same way we used to explore the fields and creek in White Lake. Now we jump out of the car and scramble up Ruby Mountain to prospect for drops of lava while Dale tells me the legend of Apache Tears. Rock hounds that we are, we delight in searching for agate and quartz and so much more. So many treasures beneath our feet!

It was Dale who taught me to track small animals and to "walk like an Indian", meaning to walk softly on the earth and with the greatest respect for nature. Together, we were one with the countryside where we lived and thrived. No longer children, we still share a respectful silence in the whispering pines and revel in the bounty and beauty that is nature. The paths we now follow are more distant and I appreciate that he continues to take pleasure in sharing time with me. Not for us the tokens and souvenirs that can be purchased in stores. Rather it is the rocks and shells and sticks and photos we collect along the way, punctuated by the conversations and values that we share.

Once he climbed a cliff to pull out a tree limb he knew I would like. I treasure it and have it still.

Always a font of knowledge, we sat beneath a large sprawling oak and he told me that one big tree like this provides enough oxygen every day for four people.

Impressive, I say.

And the same tree provides a cooling effect equal to about 5 room-sized air conditioners, he continued.

How do you know all this, I ask him? I'm smart, he replied with his familiar smirk that I love.

We had already established that he was smart. We had both taken the Mensa test. I scored 163 and he scored 165. And he never let me forget that he was the smarter one.

We had explored Colorado, New Mexico, Arizona, Texas, Mexico and the bayous of New Orleans as well as Ontario and Quebec. But there would come a time when he would take a journey on which I could not accompany him.

Ice Storm

Often, we have to trust in nature and the environment. Increasingly, nature and the environment have to trust in us. When has that relationship inspired you to live up to that trust and do more than you thought you could?

A beautiful tree, devoid of its foliage, reaches up to the sky while its roots, deep and strong, rest in the protective earth. It may appear asleep but is truly alive in its graceful, stark beauty against a winter landscape. Ahhh, the beauty of trees, in every season, inspire us with hope.

But...what will be called "The Storm of the Millennium" begins almost innocently and with no warning of what lies ahead for the beautiful trees of Eastern Ontario and Western Quebec.

According to newspaper clippings and Ottawa Hydro, our neighbourhood is worst hit within the city of Ottawa because of our many trees.

In the grip of a bizarre ice storm, a sheet of wet glass encases trees, buildings and cars in an icy shield. The night is punctuated by explosions of blue as transformers spark and sizzle and explode. Trees and limbs come crashing down. The power goes out. Live wires are everywhere. The world from my windows is chaotic.

At first it is called the Ice Storm of the Century but then it is elevated to Storm of the Millennium in terms of devastation to trees and forests not seen in past 450 years. Some areas will be out of power for over one month. Montreal, Quebec, seems to be even harder hit than Ottawa in power outages.

But we don't know this today. Today is Day One and we expect power to come back on "any minute". I light a fire in the fireplace and focus attention on my daughter, cat, the water pipes and the tree that hangs over the solarium kitchen windows. My car is locked in the garage without hydro to release it.

It is a terrible beauty. During this first night, I bear silent witness to the tinkling of ice falling around us, and of the roll, crack and crash to the earth of these wonderful old trees, friends and companions.

I shall always think of this as *"The Night the Trees Screamed."* The screams are heartbreaking. Somehow, they have warned the birds who fled and do not return for weeks. Amazing—nature's telegraphy...or telepathy.

Day Two: It is colder in the house. I stand in the freezing rain and keep the trees company. Another comes crashing down before my eyes. We hear about many that have crashed across cars and one baby that is born in a car that can't traverse the streets with downed trees. I tend fire and flame of fireplace and candles.

Day Three: Still the ice rain falls. It is breathtakingly beautiful. But the devastation is all around. A train from Ottawa to Toronto takes 18 hours with no food. Then all trains, planes and the major highway close down to Ottawa.

We are a fragile, crystal island separated from all else. My thoughts go to farmers who have cows to milk and livestock to keep alive. Word travels to the world and friends from afar call to see if we are ok. Thank heavens the phone continues to work.

Day Four: Two or more inches of ice builds up on every branch and thing that is outside. And still it falls. Tonnes of ice continue to bring down trees.

I attend meetings in Centre town where there are no trees and wires are underground. You would never know there was such devastation elsewhere. I come home, iced over myself from waiting for buses. Ours is a blackout area. It is eerie. As I get off the bus, a voice from the back says, "*You're going into a really scary area...*" I go. And it is.

The ping of ice against glass and the greyness are constant – the only companions to silence and the crackle of small flames.

Day Five: The house is now very cold. All our neighbours have moved out. I finally realize the power is not going to come on in "any minute" and have to think about survival. My daughter goes to work at a Storm Shelter. I am relieved for she will have heat, people, warm food and news through media access.

I maintain my vigil by the fire, running the little bit of water left in the pipes so they won't freeze and keeping an eye on the beautiful maple whose boughs are now heavy and groaning with ice and within an inch of the overhead solarium windows. I know I will have lost whatever food was in the fridge and freezer but it is the tree bursting through the windows that concerns me most. I move the plants and furniture away from the windows. My tree! I will it to be upright and strong enough to withstand this assault.

Day Six: Mika stays beside me in her own chair, wrapped in an afghan and fleece before the small fires. How much wood is left? Not sure. Can't see into the garage. I call some elderly friends to make sure they are being cared for. They are. I close doors to all the rooms that have them.

Even the days are dark and grey. It is eerie and hard to concentrate or write or work or sleep. By this time, over 69 ml of ice rain and 10 cm of ice pellets have fallen and ice continues to weigh down everything.

The tree touches the windows now. Mika is quiet. We are now only in the small radius in front of the fire. The wood is low. But I know my daughter is safe and warm.

10:50 p.m. – what is that sound? Can it be? Is that the furnace? The fridge? It is a moment of relief, wonderment and disbelief. I'm not sure whether to laugh or cry. It will be warm soon! There is light. Just a little. I don't want to create a surge or use too much. And I call Hydro – to say thank you. *"I know how many people's efforts it took to do this. Thank you for answering all these calls. Thank the crews who are so tired.*

152

Thank you for light and heat after all these days!" "Oh, you are giving me chills," said the woman who answered. *"Thank you so much for calling to say that!" "Good Night,"* we both say. It will be.

And soon I will stop shivering and it will be warm. We made it, Mika! We survived!

11:35 p.m. – it's gone again.

Day Seven: It comes on and stays on. My daughter comes home and sleeps after being on duty for so long. The ice rain stops and the sun comes out and so do I. To see, to touch, to listen to the whir and purr of power. What a sound – within and without! We are so lucky. There are many who will have to wait weeks before their power is restored. I also place my hands on the maple and the other trees on the big lawn. I know it is not safe to be around them yet, but I need to touch them as though in a blessing. In reverence and in thanks.

Day Eight: In the largest peacetime mobilization in Canadian history, 12,000 soldiers are sent to help in recovery from the storm. The devastation is remarkable. 150 electric transmission towers south of Montreal have been toppled as though melted into grotesque shapes. Near Ottawa, over 2,000 electrical poles had snapped like toothpicks.

It is reported that as much as 50–70% of all trees in Eastern Ontario and Western Quebec have been decimated. Some 70% of the world's supply of maple syrup comes from these areas and upstate New York. One local maple farm operator described as many as 80,000 trees were destroyed. It would take decades to rebuild. The maple syrup supply will be greatly reduced this spring.

What a year! And it's not even two weeks old yet. But I don't think I will be in a rush to set another nice fire in the fireplace or to serve a candle-lit dinner. When it is safe to do so, I stroll down streets full of broken, scarred, crippled trees and silently cry. I promise myself that one day I will work on a project that encourages our whole city, our whole country to plant one million trees. And I do.

After the Storm

I whisper to the trees. They always whisper back. Let's go for a walk, you and I. Come and meet some new friends and start your own conversation with trees. You may be so pleasantly surprised by the wisdom they will impart each time you do.

Chopping wood begins in March with the clean-up beginning in earnest as the snow melts in early April. It will take many months and, in the rural areas, years to complete. Spring also brings flooding of the Ottawa River.

The snow has covered the terrible devastation beneath it. As it melts and disappears, we are reminded of just how many and how badly our trees have been affected. The roads and streets are piled high with debris on either side. Everywhere are signs of destruction.

One large bough lies beneath an old, gnarled oak as though it has been yanked straight out with deliberate force. No wonder the trees cried and screamed that night.

I walk to the river to visit a favourite tree of mine that I have loved for many years. I want to see how it has survived the storm and the floods. The water has risen so much that it is now out in the river rather than along the edge. It is very old and looks like it might want to just topple over into the water in resignation. Poor old thing, I whisper to it. Hang on a little longer please. The flood waters will recede and your leaves will clothe you again. Soon young people (and me) will climb your outstretched limbs and birds will sing in the midst of your new life. Please don't give up yet.

Weeks later, the grass is green, the leaves provide cover for broken limbs and tree eating trucks arrive. Gives a whole new meaning to "chip trucks". I take another walk to the river. The waters have receded and leaves do clothe this wonderful old tree. The birds returned and so too, do I. It is absolutely beautiful again and I smile with delight.

Two young fellows are smoking grass nearby and they set up a conversation with me. Noticing me taking photos, one asks, *"Are you a photographer?"*
"I take pictures," I reply.

"For a newspaper?"

"No, you're safe."

"Want to take a picture of us up the tree?"

"Sure." I do and it is a terrific photo.

"Want to come up and share a toke with us?"

"Thanks, but no. Be careful."

"We will. You too!"

"I will, thanks." I wave and continue on my way, mentally blowing a kiss to the tree. You did it, old friend!

And so the journey continues, touching friends old and new along the way. Being careful, but not too careful.

Doves and Squirrels

Do you have the opportunity to interact with the creatures where you live? I hope you do. They will make you laugh. They will inspire you with their tenacity and instincts. And they will amaze you with all the life and persistence they have in their tiny selves. Time to go out and meet a new creature? Perhaps so.

A Time to Nourish, A Time to be Nourished: The Mourning Doves left a feather on my balcony. I give it to Shanty for her totem. I watch the birds scare away the big, grey squirrel. I name the squirrels. The grey must be a young Amadeus. The black with a missing ear is Vincent – Vincent van Gogh.

Another day I watch the two Mourning Doves flying and landing side-by-side on the stub of a tree where a big limb dropped out during the ice storm. It is an old tree with a big hole. Little birds fly in and out of the hole after little creatures living inside. The Doves watch. One went in. The other waits. And starts to pace. I wait too. It is now a long time that it hasn't come out. I guess it is stuck. I wonder who might have a ladder I could borrow. I wonder how to help it get out? How awful. Just what I didn't need today. But resigned to have to do something. Poor Dove.

I've been mulling over a problem. Just like the Dove, I got caught in a hole. Just like the Dove, it is of my own making.

The Dove got out. I figured out my problem. Neither of us needed a ladder.

A whole flock of yellow and black finches just moved in. How lovely. The robins are back and today one landed on my balcony while I sat there. Robins and distillfinks and doves, oh my!

A few days later, I saw the two doves walking down the road and I heard one say to the other – now don't you dare go near that hole again!

Spring progresses into summer and the remaining trees are full of birds and creatures galore. A blue jay took over my balcony and is very loud and bossy. A cardinal now lives in the kitchen maple. A chipmunk visits my window sill and shares seeds with the doves. A friend said, doves are ground feeders, they aren't supposed to eat from window sills. Well, tell them that. Two doves and the chipmunk sit side-by-side and share happily.

Summer becomes early autumn and a group of three of us have been watering and caring for the trees, grass and gardens. But the poor trees have had so much to contend with since last year's ice storm.

This summer has been so hot and now so dry that leaves are falling fast and obviously suffering.

My kitchen maple is doing well with lots of water in my small garden. But grass everywhere is browning and dry unless watered daily. Last year, the grass stayed green until mid-December but now it has been dry since August.

There was a cloudy partial lunar eclipse on August 11th from 5:55 to 6:30 a.m. Nature is affected by nature. The birds were still and only began a hesitant twittering at 6:31 a.m.

The trees on the main lawn do not look well. Especially the old one that provided a home for small insects upon which the birds could feast. But, even in its depleted state, it produced opulent mushrooms as well. And guess who claimed ownership of this decadent treat?

Why, Amadeus, of course! The crazy, grey squirrel who owns the property, or thinks he does. He is very big and fat and must be high on mushrooms as he does acrobats off the branches and twirling in the air. I've never seen such a happy, stoned squirrel! Even the tree seemed to laugh at his unique display of unknown talents.

There is such a little that trees require from us, but so much more that they contribute to everyone and everything else around them.

Tears and Petals

Strength, peace and patience – we are capable of so much more than we ever knew. We may be bruised, but not beaten. When have you been in a situation where you surpassed what you thought you could achieve? That you could give without needing recompense? Where you kept on going and giving, far beyond what you ever thought you could? This is the deep well of the spirit within us all. We may not know what is there, until we need to tap into it.

There can be opportunity in every tragedy. There can be peace in small moments. There can be triumph in small accomplishments. And there will always be grace and great beauty in the great loves of this thing called life when we share it with each other.

The blooms erupted on May 19th. It is a glorious spring day and I am looking forward to taking my Mom outside to enjoy it. It has been a long winter for both of us. After breakfast, I massage her legs with oil as I do twice every day. We do her exercises and I dress her in lovely spring colours. The hairdresser came yesterday and her white hair looks so pretty.

The Home Care woman came by for an assessment update. We talked about the wonderful young woman who comes once a week for a few hours. It is then I am able to go out for groceries, prescriptions, banking or whatever is needed. Mom loved her and I trusted her with my Mom.

As she was leaving I told her how much I appreciated the services and individuals who made it possible. She said I was doing everything possible and she wanted to help me. But you know, she said, there is a lot of deterioration since the last time.

I took her hand and guided her arm into her jacket then turned her around to do the same with the other sleeve. I suddenly stopped and we looked at each other in surprise. Margo, she said, you really have to get some respite care. I didn't even realize I had been dressing the nurse!

After lunch and pills, I guided Mom into the wheelchair Red Cross was making available to us free for three months. It went very smoothly this time. *"Mom, we're really making progress!"* She said, *"Yes, things have been going pretty well since I met you."*

I am her daughter. She has been living with me for years, but she doesn't know who I am.

I push her chair past the tree I planted for my brother, Dale. It too is showing blossoms today. I can no longer take her into the back yard to see the Colorado blue spruce, the White birches that are her favourite or the crab apple trees that are glorious. I show them to her through the windows but she can't really see them and can no longer walk out there.

But with the wheelchair, I can take her down the street and to an opening that leads to the Parkway and to the Crab Apple Orchard where we used to walk. The scents are like heaven. I wheel her right under the branches and sit on a bench beside her chair. I give her a branch of blossoms to have for her own. She looks content. Her face is reposed and relaxed.

"Do you remember being here with me before, Mom?"

She was looking straight ahead with her big, brown eyes, *"I've often tried to think of when you and I first met, but I just don't know when it was."* She doesn't know me.

Sometimes she calls me Lady or Nurse or even Daddy. I guess I am whoever she needs at the time. She is content and relaxed now but it is not always that way. She often disappears into an agitated, yelling, sleepless, demanding nightmare where I don't know her at all.

I hate these diseases that have claimed her. Parkinson's and Alzheimer Diseases have stolen the gentle, kind, loving woman that my Mom has always been and taken her to a terrible place. I am often lost and trying to understand what is happening. I go to the places she finds herself and bring her back to somewhere safe.

But this moment is a gift—a gift of time and a gift to the senses. I invite her to look up and see the lovely colours of the apple blossoms. To drink in and breathe deeply of the glorious scent that will be with us for only a short time until their time is over for this spring. To feel the warmth and wonderful light of the sun. To inhale these healing moments to the senses and to keep them within us both for all the dark times still ahead.

A gentle breeze stirs the branches above and some of the petals fall like tears around us.

Lullaby

Have you ever felt lost? Have you ever tried to help someone else who has become lost? Where do you go to find the courage and inspiration to do so? To that still small voice deep within that resides where love never gives up.

Help!!! Help!!!

Mom, where are you?!

I have to find out where she thinks she is so that I can save her.

I'm here. I'm up the tree and I can't get down!

Ok, I'm climbing up to get you. I will help you down. Don't cry.

163

She can't walk but she has climbed onto a wobbly magazine basket and holding onto the window sill where she can see the stars.

I take a firm but gentle hold of her waist and hand and gently lead her back down.

There Mom, you are safe now.

I tuck her back into bed and cover her up.

I sing her a little lullaby and she falls asleep…

At least for a little while

A Memory Garden

Have you ever planted a memory garden? If not, let's start one now. Can you imagine a special tree or plant for someone in your life? Whether they be with you now or not. Is someone a lovely rose? Is someone else a beautiful birch tree? Is there a person representing a strong oak tree in your life?

Give thought to this memory garden that you can plant in honour of those you do or have loved. Whether you plant it in the ground or just your imagination, it will stay with you forever. Enjoy the fragrance and the view. It is a gift to you and they.

As long as someone stays in our memory, they are never gone from our lives. Hold them close to your heart always even if they are no longer part of your life.

I will plant an orchard for my loved ones.
The birds will come and the creatures and insects.
A memory garden of trees.
Every tree different and every one beautiful.
Just like the people I love.

"To sit in the shade on a fine day, and look upon verdure, is the most perfect refreshment."
—Jane Austen, *Mansfield Park*

"I got a statistic for you right now. Grab your pencil, Doug. There are five billion trees in the world. I looked it up. Under every tree is a shadow, right? So, then, what makes night? I'll tell you: shadows crawling out from under five billion trees! Think of it! Shadows running around in the air, muddying the waters you might say. If only we could figure a way to keep those darn five billion shadows under those trees, we could stay up half the night, Doug, because there'd be no night!"
—Ray Bradbury, Dandelion Wine

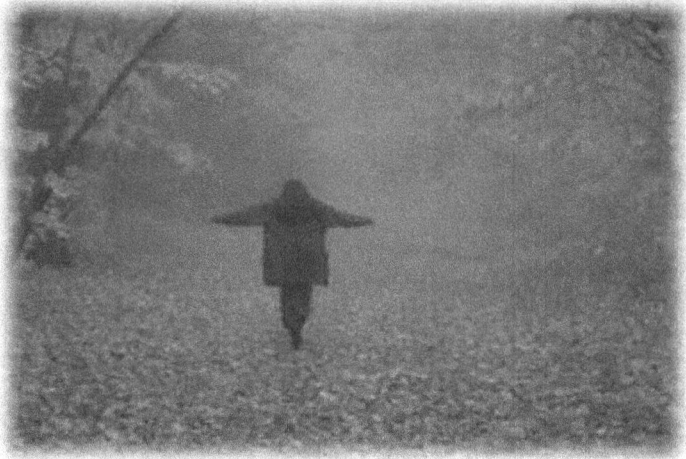

Chapter 12: What We Each Can Do

Margo Royce

"Never say there is nothing beautiful in the world anymore. There is always something to make you wonder in the shape of a tree, the trembling of a leaf."
—Albert Schweitzer

What a Mountain Pine Beetle Can Do

Kelowna, British Columbia, Canada

The mountain pine beetle is a native insect that lives most of its life under the bark of host trees. The adult spends only a few days outside of the tree while searching for a new host. Such a small creature, an adult measures only about 4 to 8 mm long, can create so much damage. Just ask the City of Kelowna in the Okanagan Valley of British Columbia, Canada.

The hills in and around Kelowna were known for their beautiful ponderosa pine forests. There were about 600,000 pines within city limits alone. They provided shade, soil stabilization, and shelter for many birds and animals year round. However, Kelowna's urban forest was hit by wildfire (the Okanagan Mountain Park fire of 2003) and then the threat of mountain pine beetles marched in. According to Provincial Government estimates, it was expected that at least 80% of all pine trees, particularly mature trees, would be lost by the year 2013.

In addition to ponderosa pine, the beetle also attacks other native and exotic pines, including Austrian, Scots, white, and lodgepole pines. Over the course of the beetle's one year life cycle, an attacked tree will start to show signs of attack as it changes color from a healthy green to yellow, then to a dark red. On the trunk of the tree there can also be evidence of the beetle in the form of frass (fine red sawdust) and/or "pitch tubes" – pitch extrusions about the size of the tip of your finger.

Beetle infested trees create safety hazards as trees are no longer wind-firm along roads, bike paths, or trails. Dead and dying trees can also increase further fire hazards, and these trees no longer provide as many environmental benefits, such as providing shade to creeks, improving air quality, or reducing storm runoff. Soil erosion may occur more frequently due to more overland flow, resulting in reduced water quality.

The mountain pine beetle presented a major challenge to the City of Kelowna because there was no guaranteed method of treatment. Infested trees were removed and destroyed to keep populations in check, but this practice was not very effective because of the huge numbers of beetles breeding in adjacent forests. There were a few treatments the city tried to use in and around Kelowna's parks for protecting individual trees or groups of high-value trees. These included the use of repellent pouches (verbenone), thinning of trees to improve their vigor ("beetle proofing"), and even an experimental treatment to wrap trees with fiberglass screening as a physical barrier against beetle attack. However, the effectiveness of these treatments seemed to vary depending upon the situation.

The last major mountain pine beetle outbreak to hit the Okanagan within recorded history was over 100 years ago. However, the most recent outbreak will likely be more severe due to past forest management practices as well as warmer winter temperatures. The City of Kelowna took a proactive approach in managing city owned forest lands in order to help limit the spread and damage. There are few markets for infested ponderosa pine, so much of the wood was ground up to make compost or provide a local sawmill where it was used to create electricity

The City of Kelowna, along with Service Canada, also developed an assistance program to help battle the pine beetle on public properties as well as assisting residential home owners to dispose of pine beetle infested wood.

In spite of the efforts of the city and private landowners, it appeared to be inevitable that most of the local pine trees would be devastated. Therefore, the city also developed plans to mount major reforestation and tree planting programs with the hope to replenish Kelowna's urban forest.

At the same time, efforts were made to guard the rest of Canada from the continued march of this intrepid beetle.

As of January, 2016, Scientists expect the beetle to continue expanding its geographic range, moving into the boreal forest and Canada's northern and eastern pine forests. They are concerned with several factors that could influence this spread.

As a normal feature of their life history, adult beetles fly to new trees and colonize. The possibility of long-distance dispersal (greater than 100 km) under favourable weather conditions is well documented.

Climate change increases suitability for infestation. Milder winters and warmer summers contribute to both higher recruitment and survival rates of the mountain pine beetle.

Susceptibility of boreal pine stands to infestation. Pine stands in the boreal forest are typically less dense and have smaller trees than British Columbia's lodgepole pine forests. Such stand characteristics may not necessarily be optimal for beetle spread, but new evidence suggests they may be less of an impediment to the spread and establishment of the beetle in boreal stands than previously believed.

Natural Resources Canada comments upon the effectiveness of forest pest management efforts, stating that control efforts now underway are reducing mountain pine beetle populations and helping to slow their speed, but the area of forest being attacked by the beetle continues to increase.

What are governments doing to slow the beetle's spread: The affected provinces and territories are leading their own beetle detection and control programs. Their efforts include detecting mountain pine beetles in new areas and removing and burning infested trees to reduce further attack, or harvesting affected stands before the economic value of the wood is lost or diminished.

Still, the boreal forest is a novel environment for this beetle and many questions—such as how quickly populations will spread and what their impact will be on forest ecological, economic and social values—have yet to be answered. Research being conducted by the Canadian Forest Service and other agencies focuses on gaining greater understanding of the ecology and population dynamics of the mountain pine beetles in the insect's new environment.

This information is being used in an ongoing risk analysis as part of the National Forest Pest Strategy, a collaboration of Canadian federal, provincial and territorial experts. The knowledge developed is assisting forest managers with assessing the threat to Canada's forests posed by the beetle and identifying effective mitigation and adaptation options.

"Man has to reconsider all traditions, all different sources, whatever facts have become available have to be reconsidered. A totally new medical approach has to be evolved which takes note of acupuncture, which takes note of ayurveda, which takes note of Greek medicine, which takes note of Delgado and his Researches—which takes note of the fact that man is not a machine. Man is a multidimensional spiritual being, and you should behave with him in the same way."
—Osho, *Medication to Meditation*

"In a forest of a hundred thousand trees, no two leaves are alike. And no two journeys along the same path are alike."
—Paulo Coelho, Aleph

"To dwellers in a wood, almost every species of tree has its voice as well as its feature."
—Thomas Hardy, *Under the Greenwood Tree*

What a School Can Do

Saskatoon, Saskatchewan, Canada

In the midst of a cold Saskatchewan winter, an educational tree planting initiative was born by the name of SPLIT, *Schools Plant Legacy In Trees*. It focused on teaching students and the community about the benefits of trees and a variety of environmental issues. The City of Saskatoon was joined by many partners including service clubs, corporate and community foundations, local contractors, nurseries and forestry staff to ensure the success and continuity of SPLIT. One elementary school a year was chosen to participate.

When a thick blanket of snow still covered the ground, thoughts about planting trees and greening school grounds and adjacent streets were well underway. Speakers came into the school to present topics including botany, ecology, soil science, insects, tree diseases and climate change. A student committee was then invited to learn about landscape design and assist with the planning and design around their school.

Students attend a Forestry Expo come spring where a variety of organizations set up interactive displays. They are provided with exposure and hands on activity about forestry and nature including pruning demonstrations by forestry workers, forestry equipment and a greenhouse tour. Every student in the school from kindergarten to grade eight participates and receives a seedling in a pot to take home as a living memory.

But still there is more! The main event is the June Planting Day at the school. Teachers, students, parents, community residents and SPLIT partners roll up their sleeves to share the big day and plant about 30 trees and 200 shrubs dependent upon the landscape plan. The day concludes with a BBQ and entertainment.

The day will end but this wonderful initiative results in improved air quality, increased wildlife habitat, shade and shelter, carbon sequestering, increased property value, beautification of the school grounds and boulevards and an enduring tree-scape for the entire community to enjoy for many years to come.

It is about five years since I first became acquainted with this beautiful, annual project as part of a Canadian Tree Challenge but I never walk by a school yard with sand and playgrounds and pavement that I don't think about this award-winning program by the city of Saskatoon, Saskatchewan, Canada.

Bravo Saskatoon! The trees will be there long after these children leave and have families of their own. Perhaps their grandchildren will one day sit beneath them and enjoy the beauty of the mature canopy. Perhaps your inspiration will touch other communities in the world to take on the environmental challenge through the education of their children while leaving a legacy of green communities and environmental stewardship.

What a gift you have given to your city, your province, your country, your children and your future... Well done, Saskatoon!

"We have nothing to fear and a great deal to learn from trees, that vigorous and pacific tribe which without stint produces strengthening essences for us, soothing balms, and in whose gracious company we spend so many cool, silent, and intimate hours."
—Marcel Proust

What a City Can Do To Recover From Dutch Elm Disease

Moncton, New Brunswick, Canada

History tells us that there were once elm-lined streets and 133 majestic elms in Moncton, New Brunswick's downtown Victoria Park. Dutch elm disease struck in the 1980s leaving only two remaining elms in Victoria Park and claiming 10,000 civic trees city-wide. Dutch elm disease is a fungal disease spread by yet another beetle – this one, the elm bark beetle that has devastated native populations of elms world-wide. Approximately one-third of Moncton's street tree population was lost to this one single pest in a lesson not soon forgotten.

The City of Moncton initiated a street planting program in the early 1990s with an annual budget of $50,000 in an effort to replace the lost urban canopy. The annual program plants over 300 40-60mm caliper trees of many varieties on City boulevards contributing to the quality of life in neighbourhoods throughout Moncton. Fifteen years later, the budget was adjusted to $100,000 in an effort to regain the original buying power that was there when the program was initiated in earlier years. The arboriculture program maintains that no more than

10% of any genus is planted to ensure there is no repeat of the effects of host specific tree pests such as Dutch elm disease. To date, 3,100 new 9'-12' deciduous trees of many types have been planted.

Tree planting is an ongoing part of Moncton's Forest Management Strategy. They also partner with the Canadian Forest Service in a Forest 2020 Project where an additional 5,000 trees are planted annually (35,000 to date) in watershed areas that demonstrate native species growth over a 20-year period.

Managing over 15,000 acres of forest land is also an important environmental program for Moncton. Local Boy Scouts planted 5-10,000 seedlings annually in watershed areas with 400,000 planted over several years. Interpretive signage demonstrates the species and year planted for outdoor education programs.

Dutch elm disease is still present in Moncton, recurring in the natural seed stock that has developed in the area and peaking every 12 – 15 years with a spike in tree mortality. Although some seed stock has regenerated over the past number of years, it is unlikely Moncton residents, and those in many other communities, will ever again see the large, graceful elms of the past.

But although thousands of majestic elms sheltering residential streets and towering over city parks is but a memory, the City of Moncton has made a determined commitment to their urban forest.

"We are the wind that carries the seeds. We are the roots of the banyan tree. We are love offered on the wing that stretches across eternity. We are a chord in life's symphony. We are the Silent Awakening!"
—Tina Malia

"I conceive that the land belongs to a vast family of which many are dead, few are living, and countless numbers are still unborn."
—Nigerian Chief

"People do not attract that which they want, but that which they are."
—James Allen

What Six Year Olds Can Do — A Class Act

Edmonton, Alberta, Canada

Unlike many areas in Canada, Edmonton has not had to deal with disease in their Elm population. In fact, it is a bigger and healthier stand than any in North America. Edmonton can also boast a protected zone of wilderness/natural parkland in the heart of the City that is the largest continuous stretch of urban parkland in North America with 7,400 hectares.

One of Edmonton's longest running programs began with the tradition of distributing evergreen seedlings to grade one students in the early 1950s as a way to celebrate Arbor Day. The Province of Alberta soon recognized the educational opportunity and stepped in to provide seedlings for every grade one student in Alberta.

Edmonton's Arbor Day is celebrated each year on the first Friday prior to May 10 with a special event in Emily Murphy Park. Close to 700 grade one students from 21 elementary schools spend a half-day at this beautiful River Valley park watching tree climbing demonstrations, riding in bucket trucks and flying on the zip line. They also learn about Forestry as a career and the importance of trees. Leading up to the day, each class receives a school visit from a city Arborist who talks about the benefits of trees, taking care of the trees in their school yards and the trees their parents and teachers received. Teachers and students alike revel in the day.

The park is full of large unique trees that have been planted to commemorate Arbor Day with two ceremonial tree plantings each year.

This event is made possible by the help of teachers, 150 parent volunteers and numerous City Parks staff and support from the Edmonton Catholic and Public School Boards. Jr. Forest Wardens get involved in the program by individually packaging the seedlings for distribution to grade ones and by planting any extra seedlings in community tree planting projects.

Alberta Sustainable Resources provided 14,000 seedlings to the City of Edmonton, and other sponsors and partners ensured the event as sustainable.

It is almost impossible to determine the number of Arbor Day trees that have been planted over the years but people from the Edmonton area, and those within Forestry Services, all remember their grade-one trees.

This program has created educational partnerships and enthusiasm within the wider community and these six year olds were not just receiving a tree but a memory and the motivation to become citizens interested in their urban canopy.

"When I am finishing a picture, I hold some God-made object up to it - a rock, a flower, the branch of a tree or my hand - as a final test. If the painting stands up beside a thing man cannot make, the painting is authentic. If there's a clash between the two, it's bad art."
—Marc Chagall

"The forest is a peculiar organism of unlimited kindness and benevolence that makes no demands for its sustenance and extends generously the products of its life activity; it provides protection to all beings, offering shade even to the axeman who destroys it."
—Gautama Buddha, 525 B.C.

"The same wind that uproots trees makes the grass shine."
—Rumi, Islamic Poet, *The Essential Rumi*

Seasons of a Tree and a Life

The time came for us to move from our home that had come to be called our Tree House. I called my daughter to let her know when I had found a new home. As I described it to her, she asked, *"Mom, will you be ok there?"* *"Yes, Honey, I'll be fine because there are mature trees outside every window."* That was important and one of the main selling features for me.

The trees and all their birds and creatures were loved. To wake at 4:30 a.m. to the joy of lustily singing birds of many varieties was a too early alarm but still made me wake with a smile for many years.

The thick foliage of the trees kept us cool in the hot summers and, as the leaves fell in late autumn, let the sun inside in the frigid winters. Both are gifts.

Last year I noticed a new little creature on my walkway. *"Well, hello! And who are you?"* Bending over to examine it, I wondered aloud, *"You must be Irish because you are such a brilliant green."*

At about the same time, I noticed that many of the trees on our streetscape were not looking their usual vibrant selves. It seemed as though parts of them were dying before my eyes.

Research taught me that the little brilliant green creature was the Emerald ash borer and that most of the trees in our extended neighbourhood were ash trees. And they were very sick.

I learned that in the early stages of an infestation, signs and symptoms are not readily apparent. This makes infestations hard to notice until numerous heavily infested dead and dying ash trees become evident. And, as I did, one might see this invasive creature strolling in our neighbourhoods at the same time as one notices the trees are dying.

I also learned the adult emerald ash borers feed on the edges of the foliage, but it is the feeding of the larvae between the bark and sapwood which results in ash tree mortality. The tree's transportation system, which moves nutrients throughout the tree and brings water up from the roots, is destroyed by the feeding of the larvae, resulting in the death of the tree by girdling.

Signs and symptoms of attack include crown dieback, bark deformities, woodpecker feeding holes, D-shaped emergence holes and shoots growing out of the trunk, roots and branches of the trees. Signs and symptoms of attack are not obvious until populations of the beetle are well established.

All of these things were certainly apparent to me after the fact. I was quite enjoying the many varieties of woodpeckers who were frequent visitors to our trees. These were all clues but I didn't put it all together until it was too late.

The adult emerald ash borer measures between 7.5 – 15 mm long. It is characterized as an Asian invasive species first detected in North America in the area of Detroit, Michigan, and later in Windsor, Ontario in 2002. It is thought that the beetle had probably been present in those areas since the early 1990s and was accidentally imported into North America via wooden packaging materials.

The beetle has proven to be highly destructive in its new range and has killed tens of millions of ash trees since its arrival. It continues to spread into new areas, with considerable economic and ecological impacts through the natural spread of the insect through flight and by the human-assisted movement of infested ash commodities (firewood, nursery stock and wood products).

Since 2005, it has continued its march across Ontario reaching the eastern edges of that province, including Canada's capital city of Ottawa, by 2013 or before. The Canadian Food Inspection Agency (CFIA) consolidated the regulated areas within Ontario and Quebec into one larger regulated area in 2014.

The National Capital Region is where we live with Canada's capital, Ottawa, on one side of the beautiful Ottawa River in Eastern Ontario and

Gatineau nestled between the other side of the Ottawa River and Gatineau Hills in Western Quebec.

Long walks on both sides of the river showed a large population of affected ash trees. An economic analysis of the impact of the loss of this population noted that many ash trees were important components of river and stream-side habitats and their loss would result in erosion of soil and change in water temperature with increased sun exposure. It further reported that gaps in the canopy of wooded areas would affect the microclimate of the forest required by some species and facilitate the invasion of exotic plant species. While ash tree loss in the urban environment would impact property values, windbreaks, temperature, pollution, runoff and the provision of homes for wildlife.

Canadian Forest Service (CFS) scientists estimate that costs for treatment, removal and replacement of trees affected by emerald ash borer in Canadian municipalities may reach $2 billion over a 30-year period.

In 2008, Gatineau, Quebec accepted a challenge to plant 100,000 trees within two years. With the enthusiasm of citizens, neighbourhood associations, community organizations and many volunteers, the city met the challenge a full year ahead of schedule.

185

But rather than resting on their laurels, the City increased their objective to 150,000 trees!

Trees contribute to the improvement of the microclimate and air quality, to the reduction of dust, carbon dioxide and urban pollution. The Gatineau program favoured planting trees in parks, school yards, public grounds and retention basins as well as along shores and roadsides. Seedlings were also distributed free to citizens along with planting tips and how to care procedures. In addition, every City councillor was given 10 mature trees to plant in their riding in the fall of 2008 and 2009.

The City had the intention of being one of the greenest cities in Quebec. A new initiative was underway as Gatineau prepared an inventory of every tree planted within its territory. Citizens were invited to enter all the trees on their property. The result would be a complete tree profile and this inventory would be compiled as a study to be used in the importance of biodiversity and in preparation of the City's tree policy. It was thought it would prove to be especially useful if an insect or other health issue attacks a certain species. It was believed to be the only inventory in the world that would represent both residential as well as municipal properties.

Well done, Gatineau, Quebec! With all of this far-sightedness and planning, the municipality was well placed to face the challenges that came in 2013 to 2016.

And the challenges came to the city and its citizens. It wasn't long before red plastic ribbons were tied around the trunks of the trees in all of our communities. I heard that some people didn't want to lose their trees on both sides of the river and were going around cutting off the red ribbons. The workers returned, of course, with red paint that couldn't be removed. Each of these tall, stately trees had received their death-knell, including all the trees that framed the homes on our street and communities.

We were told our trees would be removed the end of June, 2014. Prior to that, I went out to thank the trees for their beauty and benefits over the years and for providing homes for all the beautiful birds and creatures that inhabited them. It was saying goodbye and thank you to dear friends that would be missed.
The next morning an army of professionals arrived. Working from home, I was fascinated to watch the men booting up, strapping in, buckling up and belting in with chain saws in hand shimmying up the trees and deftly removing each bough and branch.

The dramatic sight of a man, high in the branchless tree, silhouetted against the blue sky and commencing to then cut down large pieces of the trunk from the top down. Swinging up, down and around they cut while others below took care of the tall, handsome pieces falling down. Cutting them into smaller logs, adding to chippers, discarding the leaves, they worked quickly until six trees in our immediate block were nothing but sawdust. Even the trunks were removed.

It looked terrible and was very sad. My neighbours returned one by one at end of afternoon and all stopped with mouth agape and eyes wide in disbelief and wonder turning to sadness – trying to take in the scene before entering their homes. One neighbour came around the corner and just stopped in horror, unable to continue walking for several moments. *"I knew they were doing it today,"* she said, *"but I wasn't prepared for what it would look like or how it would affect me."*

We knew that saplings would be planted in their places but it would take thirty years for them to grow. We knew it would never be the same again. And it isn't. The new plantings took place in October of 2014. In spring of 2015, all the remaining trees in the back of our property were also removed. They were not replaced. The song birds have left. And if we waken at an early hour, it is only to be greeted by silence.

Sometimes the people and places we love remain in our hearts but are no longer in our lives.

We must never miss an opportunity to celebrate, honour and love those who are still with us. And to honour them in our memory when they are no longer in our lives.

Sometimes we lose the people we love, the homes we love, the trees we love. But we tuck their memories into our hearts and keep going with their beauty and strength as the gifts we carry forward. Because we must.

And we plant a tree in their memory.

And sometimes the birds return anyway. The beautiful, cheeky, acrobatic chickadees frolic on the bird feeders. Robins have to sing even without a tree. Cardinals visit and the bossy blue jays come in numbers to our Blue Spruce and Pines. The clever crows caw their greetings. I have even been visited by a Bald Eagle and a very special Eurasian Collared Dove who is not supposed to be in this region has adopted me. The geese fly overheard and ducks waddle by. Seagulls squawk...

And the trees will grow...

And the trees will grow

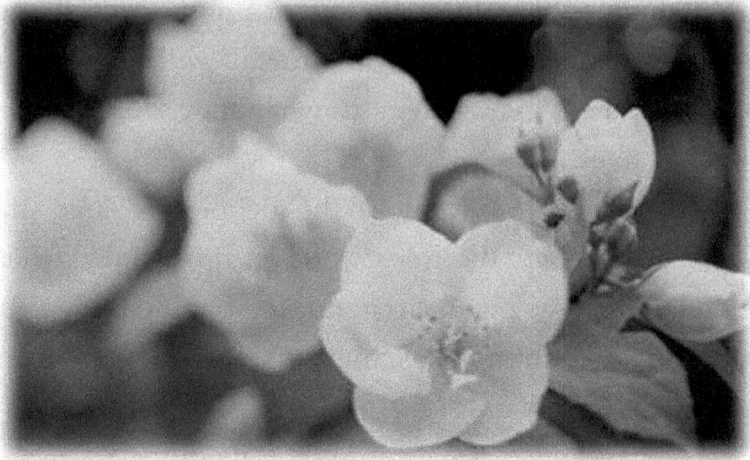

Chapter 13: Trees, Body Parts, and Unity

Kimberly Burnham

Here are some poems, written by Kimberly Burnham, based on the work of Avia Venelica. When you consider the energy of each of the parts of the tree, which do you most identify with or resonate with? From which part of the tree do you want draw more energy or strength? Can you draw vitality from leaves, generosity from branches, or stability or growth from the heartwood? Can a tree's roots teach you to reach for what nourishes you? As you read, feel the energy and symbolism in the words. Do they resonate for you? What do they change in your body or your mind?

"By hanging out in the branches of tree symbolism we can derive fathoms of higher understanding. This is what Ecointuition is all about: Moving our illumined perception into the deeper realms of Nature with a focus on gaining insight - even enlightenment. Trees are uniquely positioned to extend these gifts of enlightened knowledge. They are timekeepers. They are wisdomkeepers. When unfurled in their luscious glory, leaves express themselves in a myriad of colors. Most predominantly however, they reveal themselves in viridian greens—a color notorious for healing, abundance, and vitality in life. When I think of green, my mind moves into Anahata energy—the realm of the heart chakra, which deals with inclusion, love, empathy, wealth, health and a whole slew of other marvelous attributes. Draw green into your own awareness and see if you settle into a sense of opulence, health and luxury."

—Avia Venefica *Ecointuiting Tree Symbolism* www.Tokenrock.com/articles/ecointuiting-tree-symbolism-127.html

Unfurled Leaves

A myriad of colors
unfurled in luscious glory
leaves revealing themselves
verdant greens
healing heart
flowing along leafy veins
like a tiny trunk with branches
liver and gallbladder meridians
notorious abundance
vitality in life
unfurl yourself
with inclusion, love,
empathy, wealth, health
inner vision
oxygen breathing out from the leaves
carbon dioxide flowing in
opulence, health and luxury

"Life is symbolic. Start interpreting."
—Avia Venefica

Abundant Branches

Trees are never
about limitation
branches express a diverse focus
generous geometry
ever-extending
reaching out
for more
of what is desired

Trees seek an abundance of light
freedom nourishing
awareness
reaching skyward
towards the blue sunlight

Amazingly nimble
growing in gravity-defying contortions
always into no limits
life depends on expansion
around obstacles

Trees teaching
there is always another way

Tough Exterior Trunk

Incredible design
outer bark protects
the whole
shielding from harsh realities

Intricate inside
fragile spirals
energetic flow
trees renewed from the inside out
sacred wisdom passed
from tree
to humankind
will you share it back again

Renewal must first be
active
growing from within

Heartwood

Centermost pillar of stability
heartwood
the trunk of a tree
center core supports
the entire system
biological reproductive stillness
inner emptiness
singing vessel
an open heart
empties out
stands strong and tall
from the inside out

*"Did you ever find a fairy near some budding little
thickets.
And when she sees you creeping up to get a closer peek
She tumbles through the daffodils, a playing hide and seek."*
—Marjorie Barrows

*"If the foot of the trees were not tied to earth, they would be
pursuing me.. For I have blossomed so much, I am the envy
of the gardens."*
—Rumi, Islamic poet

Deep Roots

Anchors, gripping tightly
to home
Mother Earth's symbiotic union
earth gives freely
nutrients and water
spanning miraculous lengths
of time and space
ever reaching
sharing healing nourishment

Dig deep be firmly rooted
think happy thoughts
grow above and below
be reflective
upward mobility
allowing for a sway above

Hidden from view
unseen by the common eye
growth and power
occurs
beneath superficial layers

Beliefs, sacred, and scared
anchor us in our lives

inner growth evident
in the outer world
radiate outwardly from the inner light

"Aromatherapy is extremely useful. If you want to go to sleep at night, and you have an aroma that calms your mind, it will help you sleep."
—Deepak Chopra

"A tree is a self: it is 'unseen shaping' more than it is leaves or bark, roots or cellulose or fruit ... What this means is that we must address trees as we must address all things, confronting them in the awareness that we are in the presence of numinous mystery."
—Brian Swimme, mathematical cosmologist,
The Universe is a Green Dragon

"In the eyes of a seer, every leaf of a tree is a page of the Holy Book and contains divine revelation ..."
—Hazrat Inayat Khan, Sufi teacher

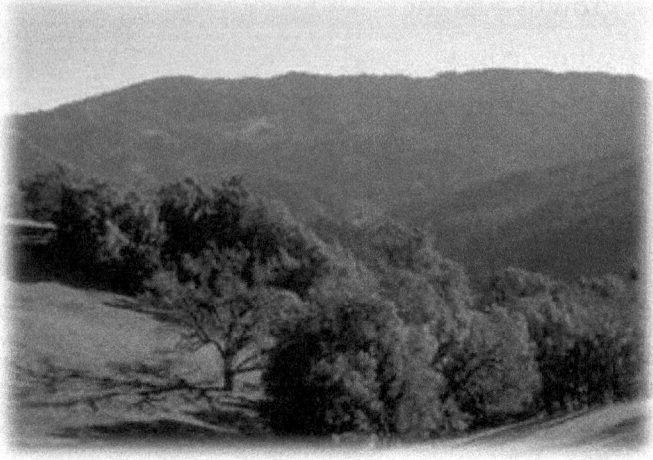

Chapter 14: Trees and Levels of Healing

Daniel Tigner (Hafiz)

Here are some of the correlations between the body of a tree and human psychology. Which level do you feel most attuned to? Spend some time meditating on the bough or trunk of a tree. Does it change your level of awareness of the opportunities around you? Does it change how you feel as you interact with other people? Notice what changes when you connect to a particular part of a tree.

Bough—Level 5 (Self, Pure Awareness)— Bliss Body

Higher consciousness, the sky, the purest level of resonance

Healing through: Meditation, Witnessing and watchfulness...

Leaves—Level 4 (Awareness, Reflection)—Body of Consciousness. Mental Body

The effect of thinking, beliefs and programming on health.

Healing through: Hypnosis, Dialogue, Contemplation...

Flowers and Fruit—Level 3 (Vibration, Resonance)—Feeling Body

Subtle energy, the effect of moods, emotions, and resonance on our well being

Healing through: Homeopathy, Music and Vibrational Tree and Flower Essences...

Trunk–Level 2 (Aura, Life Force)– Etheric Body

The effects of the flow of energy, Chi, and the Circulation of energy on our health.

Healing through: Prana breathing, Dance, Qui Gong, Yoga, Acupuncture. Walks in the woods, Nature, the etheric energy of trees…

Roots–Level 1 (Chemistry)–Physical Body

The effects of diet, nutrition, hygiene, physical environment, genes and constitution on our health.

Healing through: Western medicine, drugs, surgery, herbs, naturopathy, cleansings, exercise…

Many healing systems work on more than one level such as Ayurvedic medicine, the ancient healing system of India. Being with trees and nature we attune to all five levels of healing and well being - Optimum health happens when we resonate at all these levels.

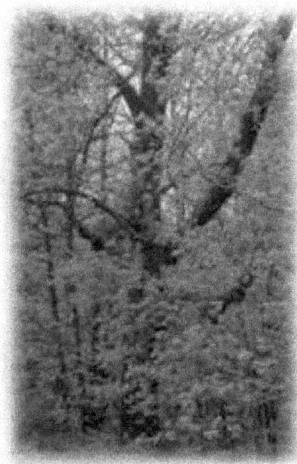

Chapter 15: Trees and Human Personalities

Kimberly Burnham

Read the following poems written by Kimberly Burnham. Is there one that stands out for you as being related to the way you look at life? Are you more like a seed or a spice or some other part of the tree? Do you want to be more like the bark or more like the flower? What can you learn from this way of looking at trees? Bring out your true character more fully. Consider how these poems can help you be more true to yourself and the dreams you have for your life.

"The Fragrant Mind falls into three parts. Part One presents a fascinating background to the subject, and explains how essential oils work on the brain. Part Two explains how essential oils can enhance emotional well-being and promote positive feelings, and includes a practical A-Z section which advises on a wide range of emotional problems, from stress and depression to moodiness and insomnia. Part Three introduces a whole new concept in aromatherapy - personality enhancement - and explains the particular characteristics of individual essential oils and how they can be matched to human personality types. You can find out, for example, whether you are a Floral, Herbie, Rootie, Woodie, Fruitie or Seedie type, and create your own tailor-made personality blends."

—Valerie Ann Worwood is internationally acknowledged as one of the world's leading aromatherapists and is the author of the bestselling *The Fragrant Pharmacy, The Fragrant Mind and The Fragrant Heavens*. These poems come out of working with her in a class.

"When Jean Valnet, MD, ran out of antibiotics during World War II, he discovered that eucalyptus oil was effective in killing almost three-quarters of staph bacteria in the air. You, too, can squash bacteria with this powerful essential oil: if you're beginning to catch a cold, try inhaling steam from a basin filled with hot water and a few drops of eucalyptus essential oil. You may just stop that cold in its tracks. Some of the most powerful antiseptic essential oils include lavender oil, tea tree oil, and clove oil."

—Althea Press, *Essential Oils for Beginners: The Guide to Get Started with Essential Oils and Aromatherapy*

"What we are doing to the forests of the world is but a mirror reflection of what we are doing to ourselves and to one another."

—Mahatma Gandhi

"A tree is like a saint. It calls no one to itself, nor does it send anyone away. It offers to protect everyone who wants to come to it, whether this be a man, a woman, a child, or an animal."

—Ma Anandamayi Ma, Indian saint.

Tree Flowers of the World

Creating a mood
all by themselves
conveying the essence
a season dressed in their flowers

Purple, pink and white
early and late
huge tulip blossoms
tiny fig tree flora

Flirtaceous and sensual
loving a good romance
strive to attract
those giving connection

Crave attention
power and status
achieve themselves
attach to someone powerful

Fashionably attractive
fun-loving, follow the trends
keep up with appearances

Thriving on being
desirable
superficial, sensitive
soft-hearted

Objects of jealousy
much misunderstood
turn it around
find understanding

"Aromachology is a term that was first coined by the Fragrance Foundation's research and education division, the Sense of Smell Institute. Although the two fields have similarities, aromachology deals specifically with the psychology of fragrance, taking a scientific approach to the relationship between fragrance and the mind."
—Vetiver Aromatics

"The human sense of smell is about ten thousand times more powerful than other senses, and scent travels to the brain so rapidly that the mental or physical response to the fragrance an essential oil emits can be immediate."
—Althea Press, *Essential Oils for Beginners*

Sweetness of Fruit

Futility of comparing
apples to oranges
hazelnuts and pinenuts
designed to nourish
someone

Is fruit
self-aware and emotionally balanced
hard workers
striving to please
great pleasure
in a job well done
millions nourished

Industrious in work
playful and benevolent
small in number those we call true friends
devoting so much
to those inner circle beings
friends for life
first to offer encouragement

Homebody Herbs

Herbies proud
and drawn to home
loving family
finding fulfillment
taking care of those closest

Like salt of the earth
flavor of life
hard work
brings out the best

Solid and dependable,
helping hands
good neighbors
calm uneventful lives
happy to be
hearing about the exploits
of others
thrive on knowing
what's goes on

Leafing Out

Leafies are the intellectuals
a world of deep love for learning
at home in research classrooms
a library

Introspective and solitary
even detached
idealistic and political at the edge
thriving on a good debate
quick to see
expanding horizons
broad perspectives
stepping back
to take in big pictures

Making connections
between seemingly unrelated
events and facts.
leafies are innovative
ideas blazing

Stalwart Resinies

The sticky stuff of life
resinies are moral stalwarts
proud to be
hard working along the path
spiritual purity
high goals
a life of principle
interested in the state of the world

Feeling
the world in a moral decline
work ethic
volunteering
charitable
strong will

Sturdy foundations
weather hardship
with ease and faith
hold on
faithful

Laidback Rooties

Easy going rooties
laidback
exude a stability
serenity
putting others at ease
a deep love
tradition and convention
quiet modest life

Peacefulness and tranquility
shying away from a fight
mistaken for weak
glossing over problems
composed and controlled
firmly grounded
dedicated toward peace
conflict mediators par excellence

"A person is made up of a Mind, a Body and a Spirit, rather than these being separate they are always influencing the others."
—Elizabeth Ashley, *The Complete Guide To Clinical Aromatherapy and Essential Oils of The Physical Body: Essential Oils for Beginners*

Seed Dreamers

Creative spirits
seedies thrive on beauty
finding wonder in the most
mundane experiences

Beauty everyday
keen observational powers
vivid memories
powerful intuition

Empaths
tuned into needs
motivation intuitions
others' and own
dreamy creators
reinventing themselves
on a regular basis

New styles,
new jobs, new religions
see what "fits" best
self assured individuals

Exhilarating Spices

Spices' fascination
feeling good
joyously, exhilarating, animated
animated adventures
dynamic go-getters

Excellent entrepreneurs
love of the high life
days at the stores
nights on the town
not for status
seeking rather love
and new experience

Deciduous all spice and cloves
pepper corns
chocolaty carob
cinnamon and nutmeg

Trendsetters without trying
naturally drawing others
vital debonair personality

Strong Wood

Independent ethical
strong woodie are
compassionate, and dedicated

Find the cause
leaning in
nuanced textured support
determined to have an impact

Power not for the status
woodies dream
ability into the shape
of the world
seeking out injustice

Making the world
a better place
loving nature
find ways to experience
the outdoors
camping,
boating
or golfing for a cause

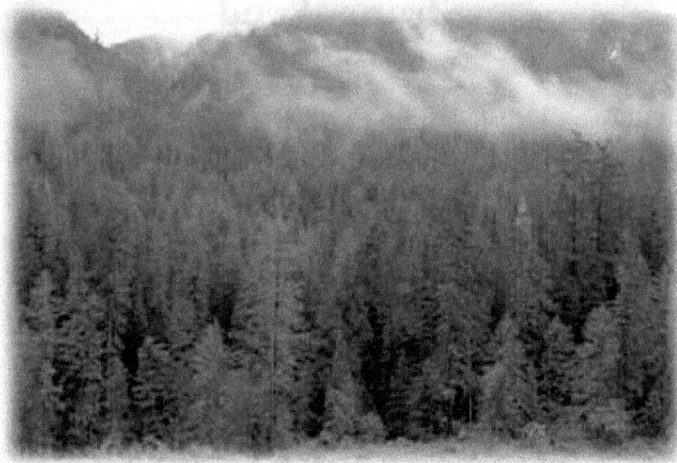

Chapter 16: Heart to Heart

Céline Cloutier (Gulabo)

Use these consciousness exercises from Céline Cloutier (Gulabo) to see and take the steps you need to reach your greatest goals and aspirations. She explains how each of five trees can influence your contemplations and approaches in each exercise.

Contemplate the Small Leaf Linden tree along with the statement, *"We are neither our thoughts nor the sensation we experience."*

Contemplate the White Trillium along with the statement, *"I am love."*

Contemplate the Yoshino Cherry along with the statement, *"I am grace."*

Contemplate the Banyan along with the statement, *"I am."*

Contemplate the Yellow Birch along with the statement, *"Calmness is my true nature."*

"Love is the secret key; it opens all the locks. The master key...."
—Osho, *The Path of Love – Discourses on Songs of Kabir*

Emotions: the Movement of Feeling

Emotions: From mind to emotions - such as impatience arising for doing this silly exercise - remember, just watch, and return your attention to breathing. Don't mind emotions either.

Before you begin these meditations take a moment and answer for yourself:

Are you the body? Yes or no.

Are you the mind? Yes or no.

Are you emotions? Yes or no.

If your answer is yes to one of all of them, ask yourself why you think you are. If your answer was

215

no to all of them, ask yourself, If not the body-mind-emotion, then Who am I?

Do this simple meditation daily if you can. Instantly or gradually you may start getting glimpses of that experience of who you are as it is awaiting to be recognized. You will certainly experience silence between two breaths as you exhale, and just before you inhale again. Take time to notice. Or as you meditate regularly, you may find yourself, nowhere, no body, no thoughts. You may come back and say, where was I? As you meditate for 5, 10, 15 minutes or more, let yourself fall into that nothingness space. Do not anticipate, do not judge, just enjoy a time of rest and peace!

"Someone is sitting in the shade today because someone planted a tree a long time ago."
—Warren Buffett

"If you deconstruct Greece, you will in the end see an olive tree, a grapevine, and a boat remain. That is, with as much, you reconstruct her."
—Odysseas Elytis

Exercise #1 How Are You?

When I meet with people in search of answers, this is what happens.

I first ask, *"How are you?"* This is a polite question often used rapidly as we walk by someone we know at the bank or the grocery store, and we hardly have time to listen to the answer.

But in a *Heart to Heart* session it is quite valuable. The first 5 minutes creates the opportunity to take the pulse, and see what seems to be most important in the moment. The picture revealed of the outside world from this person, often reflects an inner state. And besides that, we, as human beings, need to communicate, to be heard, and share.

First step: Go ahead and ask yourself: How am I? How do I feel right now about my life? What is bothering me? What is missing?

These simple questions help reveal to one self what seems to be the issues in the way of experiencing truth and happiness. Once out in the open, work can begin. Cleaning the cupboards helps see what is at the bottom.

Second Step: answer the following: If you had 3 wishes, what would they be? Everything is eligible. For example; feeling peaceful, sleep, stop being afraid all the time, money, a relationship, a new house ...

Third Step: look at what is stopping you from achieving those goals.

Have you ever tried to improve yourself? Does it work? Think of resolutions you take on the 1st of January each year: lose weight, be more patient, get my house organised, take more time for myself, meditate, eat healthier, etc. etc. etc.

Look at the steps taken, and how gradually you lost sight of your great intentions, resolutions, goals, way of living, etc.

TREE to contemplate: Small Leaf Linden (*Tilia cordata* and cultivars).

Nourishes and expands: This tree offers protection and clearing of thoughts and impressions. Its resonance helps create a space of light around us. Clarity arises between, one's own thoughts and information that is extraneous.

Brings awareness and resolution to: As we pick up all sorts of information and unwanted thoughts we become vulnerable. It is easy to get hooked by outside influences and it becomes hard to decipher what is ours, and what arises from our own experiences and insights. We become full of a chattering traffic of thoughts.

218

Contemplation: We are neither our thoughts nor the sensation we experience.

Tree essence: This tree can be found in Therapist Healer Essence and Aura Cleansing Spray.

"My experience is that changes in resonance become perceptible after about a three-month period. Growth in resonance is like growth in meditation. It happens very slowly, unnoticeably. Perhaps you could compare the growth rate of resonance with that of trees. If you look at a tree regularly to see if it is growing, you become discouraged - it always looks the same. But if you forget about it, live your life, and one day by chance walk past that tree again, you suddenly realize it is bigger than the last time you saw it."
—Ma Sagarpriya, *The Master's Touch - Psychic Massage*

"Nature's peace will flow into you as sunshine flows into trees. The winds will blow their own freshness into you, and the storms their energy, while cares will drop off like autumn leaves."
—John Muir, *Our National Parks*

Exercise #2 The Level of the Mind

Why don't efforts to improve work? Maybe, it is because your efforts remain on the level of the mind and you are going against a mastermind, who has all the tricks in the books to keep you the same, to keep you in what is known and familiar. One thing to remember, *transformation occurs at the level of the heart.*

As we grew up - and for most of our life - we learned to move away from our spontaneity, because we bothered people with our energy. We began doubting our intuition as our choices were judged and disapproved. We became a stranger to our heart, because along the way we may have gotten hurt badly and lost faith. All of this translated into our losing sight of our True Self.

A spring flower found under trees to contemplate: White Trillium (*Trillium grandiflorum*)

Nourishes and expands: Purity of heart is experienced with White Trillium. It soothes and heals. We can simply be ourselves and we sense no need to compare ourselves with other. Its energy is like spring, revitalizing at many levels.

Brings awareness and resolution to: Wounds of the heart, feeling of burden. We lack self-esteem; we imagine ourselves to be lacking, no matter what. We compare ourselves to others.

Contemplation: I am Love.

Tree Essences: This tree can be found in Healing the Heart Essence and Spray.

"I went to the springs while the sun was still up, and sitting on a rocky outcrop above the cave mouth I watched the light grow reddish across the misty pools, and listened to the troubled voice of the water. After a while I moved farther up the hill, where I could hear birds singing near and far in the silence of the trees. The presence of the trees was very strong...The big oaks stood so many, so massive in their other life, in their deep, rooted silence: the awe of them came on me, the religion."
—Ursula K. Le Guin, *Lavinia*

"These people have learned not from books, but in the fields, in the wood, on the river bank. Their teachers have been the birds themselves, when they sang to them, the sun when it left a glow of crimson behind it at setting, the very trees, and wild herbs."
—Anton Chekhov, "A Day in the Country"

Exercise #3 The Impostor

Life is a multitude of experiences from all senses. We see, hear, taste, touch and feel and, we, as multilevel beings, rapidly accumulate thousands of vibrations and impressions. To make sense of all this information, and of each experience, our good mind decided it had to organize our life and make rules for survival. To do so, we invented *the Imposter,* a sort of a puppet-master in and over me.

On the outside, we may live our life as though everything is fine. When asked, *"How are you?"* We reply, *"I am great and you?"*

We work, we buy a house, we get into relationships, raise children, do our best to fit into this civilization and, if there are crises, we have developed mechanisms to cope and keep order. It may work for a certain time, until one day, we feel lonely, depressed, angry, sad, envious, and mostly empty. At that point, if we were to ask ourselves, *"Who am I,"* we would not know. To this question, we might fill up pages of labels, images, and roles we play in our life, but our true identity has been buried and access shut down.

Why? Because that seems to be how being human works. We seem to be masters at making a mess of things. We become slaves of the rules we created and live our lives to fit in, to avoid facing our self and to survive. We have been so busy trying to do, improve, fix, please and follow rules, our mind is infinitely filled with garbage. No wonder we cannot hear God's whisper anymore.

Good news! There is true hope! Your True Self is alive and present, because we are vibration, we are light, we are a pulse of love, and this beautiful being is as close as your next breath.

One has to take time daily to practice going into the heart, sitting in silence, so we can hear again the natural pulse, and regain faith in reclaiming our birthright, forgotten along the way, and, kick that stranger, *the Imposter*, out.

TREE to contemplate: Yoshino Cherry (*Prunus x yedoensis*)

Nourishes and expands: Cheerfulness. A profound antidote for fear. Receiving grace. This tree reminds us of our ultimate Buddhahood and enlightenment. It recalls the story of Buddha sitting beneath a tree showering its flowers upon him. Blessings, compassion, kindness, grace and love raining on us.

Brings awareness and resolution to: Fear of all sorts. Feeling confused, ungrounded and not knowing where to turn. Desperation.

Contemplation: I am grace.

Tree Essence: Yoshino Cherry is found in the Light Essence.

"Until then, have great expectations. Keep believing you dreams will come true. And remember, when life throws you a pit... plant a cherry tree."
—Coleen Murtagh Paratore, *The Wedding Planner's Daughter*

"What a pity every child couldn't learn to read under a willow tree..."
—Elizabeth George Speare, *The Witch of Blackbird Pond*

"In the spring, at the end of the day, you should smell like dirt."
—Margaret Atwood, *Bluebeard's Egg*

Exercise #4 Time to Stop!

It is time to stop.

Fourth Step: Sit - somewhere comfortably, nothing fancy about your position, put on a gentle music if you wish as it may help to Relax and occupy the mind.

Begin: Take a deep breath, exhale. Take another one, very deep, exhale. One more time, relax.

Body: Go from toes to top of head and send a conscious intention to each body part to relax.

Breathing: Start becoming aware of your breath pattern. This is a natural happening since birth, you have nothing to do. Just BE the witness of your own breath. Let it be natural.

Mind: As it thinks it is in control, it will want your attention, just like a little kid. Do not mind the mind. Keep your attention on your breath. Follow it. If the mind gets to you, gently return to your breath. That is the only effort.

Tree to Contemplate: Banyan (*Ficus benghalensis*)

Nourishes and expands: Banyan helps the growth of pure awareness, the remembrance of "Who I am." A tree that helps with direct inquiry into self. We touch the unmovable and silent center of being.

225

Brings awareness and resolutions to: Lack of awareness, disconnected from our inner being. The roots growing from the tree are like the various tendencies of mind and endless thoughts.

Contemplation: I am.

Tree Essence: This tree can be found in Light essence and Self Awareness spray.

"Do you know that even when you look at a tree and say, `That is an oak tree', or `that is a banyan tree', the naming of the tree, which is botanical knowledge, has so conditioned your mind that the word comes between you and actually seeing the tree? To come in contact with the tree you have to put your hand on it and the word will not help you to touch it."

—Jiddu Krishnamurti, *Freedom from the Known*

"Should you shield the canyons from the windstorms you would never see the true beauty of their carvings."

—Elisabeth Kübler-Ross

Exercise #5 Doing Nothing

For most people the most difficult thing to do is nothing. Meditation is really doing nothing, expecting nothing, changing nothing. That is why most people do not stick to it. Comments I hear are about restlessness in the body and too many thoughts, and feeling inadequate. Of course, it is the mind's job to keep us occupied!

Imagine you are going to a football game, or a play, or a ballet. You are a guest; you are invited to just watch the show. Do you step into the stage? NO. Then do the same in meditation. Sit back, observe the scene and learn about what you have become. Watch the body, watch the mind and emotions in order to observe how *the Imposter* has learned to operate. Sit still. Only when you vanquish this stranger, will your real identity reveal itself to become the true master.

Tree to Contemplate: Yellow Birch (*Betula alleghaniensis*)

Nourishes and expands: You begin to feel the silence and emptiness as a rich musical experience. Welcoming moments of stillness. Becoming receptive to experience oneness with all.

Brings awareness and resolution to: Fear of darkness, emptiness. Escaping the moment, stillness. Tendency of always being occupied.

Tree Essence: This tree can be found in the single essence called Relaxation (Yellow Birch)

Contemplation: Calmness is my true nature.

"I'd like to go by climbing a birch tree~
And climb black branches up a snow-white trunk
Toward heaven, till the tree could bear no more,
But dipped its top and set me down again.
That would be good both going and coming back.
One could do worse than be a swinger of birches."
—Robert Frost

"A shaft of moonlight illuminated a row of sentinel silver birch in a phosphorescent glow, appearing almost ethereal in the relative surrounding gloom. Boris had stopped again, his silhouette a stark black juxtaposition against the background of illuminated branches."
—R.D. Ronald, *The Elephant Tree*

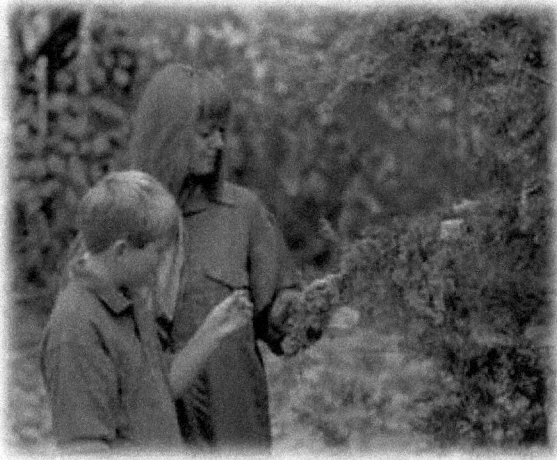

Chapter 17: The Principle of Resonance

Daniel Tigner (Hafiz)

If a gong is struck and then a second gong, their sounds will reverberate or resonate together producing a richer and deeper tone. If you were to hum you would find yourself resonating easily to that sound, your voice taking on a deep timber. You might even feel that resonance vibrating in areas of your body. Daniel Tigner (Hafiz) asks us to pay attention to the sounds around us, particularly the natural sounds.

Sound demonstrates clearly the principle of resonance, but it is not only sound that resonates through us but moods, feelings and more interior spaces as well. Take for example the infectious excitement of fans at a hockey game or in a cinema tears rolling down the cheeks of the audience, waves of emotions, as they watch the story of lovers parting forever from each other. Holding hands with a friend as we walk through the woods we are enveloped in a mellow mood of quietude and beauty. This is what happens when many people meditate together. There is the resonance of silence and serenity.

As we become more aware of resonance we will note that certain parts of us feel resonant and responsive, while other areas seem denser, heavier. We may for example feel aliveness in our hands or heart, but have little contact with our legs.

The most important way the agents of healing support us is through their resonance, nourishing areas of resonance within ourselves. For example, ingesting a vibrational tree essence nurtures our resonance. It is like giving water to a tree so that it may grow.

Resonance is that underlying quality of vitality and pleasure experienced when we appreciate beauty, feel warmth in the presence of a friend, expand in love or are moved by music.

Resonance is the core of the healing experience. We sometimes may need to confront problems, use therapy to help us to uncover, release wounds or to give us space to understand better, but if there is no resonance growing, there can be little deep healing. Therapy can help clear the path, but simply to work on problems, as if we were a problem, or as if our so-called problems could be solved if we somehow corrected our faults, is not an attitude that engenders deeper healing. There needs to be an expansion, a growth in our aliveness and awareness.

"It is quite affecting to observe how much the olive tree is to the country people. Its fruit supplies them with food, medicine and light; its leaves, winter fodder for the goats and sheep; it is their shelter from the heat and its branches and roots supply them with firewood. The olive tree is the peasant's all-in-all."
—Fredrika Bremer

"One will never again look at a birch tree, after the Robert Frost poem, in exactly the same way."
—Paul Muldoon

Attention Is Food

This is a fundamental principal. There are probably few things as painful as being ignored. If a child is ignored he fades; loving attention is the garden in which a person flowers. Attention is such a deep need that children seek it whether through positive means or by creating difficulties. Whatever we nourish expands. *"Love begets love"* and *"hate begets hate."* If we nourish our sense of beauty, love or strength, those qualities that make us more whole, empower us, we feel more alive.

Trees have a nourishing presence. As trees share their light they nourish our own resonance thereby supporting and empowering us on our healing journey.

"In this world hate never yet dispelled hate. Only love dispels hate. This is the law, Ancient and inexhaustible."
—Gautama the Buddha, *The Dhammapada*

"Adopt the pace of nature: her secret is patience."
—Ralph Waldo Emerson

The Effect of Expanding Resonance

What is nourished expands and grows in us.

Over the longer term it is the expansion of resonance that is healing. One of the great things about being with a tree that we feel a strong affinity with is that it nurtures our resonance. Trees are wonderful as they don't judge us. We can relax and simply be there, present – and that is a great gift!

Resonance starts with what is right: what is alive and flowing and then continues to nourish it. Nourish yourself with good things (thoughts and feelings included) every day.

Resonance honors and appreciates self.

Resonance does not force change.

Resonance does not condemn you. It is contradictory to expand love for oneself or others, if the starting point is self-condemnation.

By expanding resonance the inner light of awareness grows.

Consciousness is brought to unconscious patterns and conditionings where they can be released and transformed through understanding.

Resonance is embracing oneself, is moment to moment, rejecting nothing. This takes courage, but it is deeply healing, allowing energy previously used to repress awareness of what we consider undesirable qualities to be freed for the growth of resonance.

In our lives, we want to clear the path of obstacles, allow resonance to grow, as that expansion of resonance is healing.

"Our future is our children; the future of the world is in their hands and in the hands of their children. Let us train them wisely, and see that the understanding and appreciation of trees is part of their heritage."
—Richard St. Barbe Baker, *Man of the Trees*

"People say that what we're all seeking is a meaning for life. I don't think that's what we're really seeking. I think that what we're seeking is an experience of being alive, so that our life experiences on the purely physical plane will have resonances with our own innermost being and reality, so that we actually feel the rapture of being alive."
—Joseph Campbell, *The Power of Myth*

Things to Do to Support the Expansion of Resonance

"Chance: I like to watch the young plants grow.
Eve: It is wonderful, isn't it?
Chance: Young plants do much better if a person helps them."
—Jerry Kosinski and Robert C. Jones, Screenplay for the movie *Being There*

"I'm an old man and have known a great many troubles, but most of them have never happened."
—Mark Twain, quoted from *Bush Flower Essences*, Ian White

Find out where you are resonant and help this to grow.

Nourish the light in you.

Make friends with a tree.

At the heart of resonance is meditation, which means to be here now in a state of alertness. It is a coming home to oneself, a residing in ones center. This is nourished in formal meditation practices, amongst which are a number of beautiful tree meditations. Set some time each day to be simply with one Self.

Resonance is the ground, the foundation of healing. On this basis, you may use therapies, medicines, etc. to help heal wounds, blocks to a fuller resonance.

Go back over your life and recall those moments that you treasure. Explore them. Feel them. Collect them. Amongst these may be transcendent or peak moments. Note what happened inside of you.

Notice moments of satisfaction and other tastes of resonance you have every day. It can be as simple as being touched by a smile.

Choose those things that nourish resonance: enjoyable activities, aesthetically pleasing things, friendliness, good food and exercise.

Listen, feel, pay attention to that which nourishes you and move away from that which is non-resonant.

Trust your higher consciousness to guide you, beginning first with little things.

"I looked at my hands to see if I was the same person. There was such a glory over everything. The sun came up like gold through the trees, and I felt like I was in heaven."
—Harriet Tubman

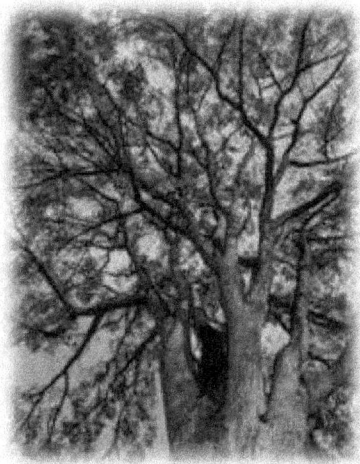

Chapter 18: Can We Communicate With Trees?

Daniel Tigner (Hafiz)

Do trees have a language, a form of intelligence, even self-awareness? Do they feel anything akin to emotion? Are they perhaps even aware of our presence and respond or attempt to communicate with us in certain ways?

In *The Consciousness of Trees*, a film by Dan McKinney, Suzanne Simard, a forester and professor at the University of British Columbia, Canada, shows that all trees in a forest ecosystem are interconnected.

The oldest and largest tree standing is thought of as a mother tree as it roots extent out far, reaching to many other trees. The trees form a kind of a communications network, with the mother tree at the center of the hub.

"My research does show that they (trees) are communicating. Yes, it's a method of communication... These plants are not really individuals in the sense that Darwin thought they were individuals competing for survival of the fittest. In fact, they are interacting with each other, trying to help each other survive," says Professor Simard.

Her work provides evidence that the practice of clear cutting, which removes the oldest mother trees, may be destructive to the forest.

In a Ted Talk entitled "The Roots of Plant intelligence," Italian researcher, Stefano Mancuso, outlines possibilities of using plant root systems in computing. Plants may indeed have a brain with a vast neural network, something like a plant internet. Does that mean true intelligence and self-awareness? – the idea is exciting and, seemingly not so farfetched.

So we studied the root apex and we found that there is a specific region that is here, depicted in blue - - that is called the "transition zone." And this region, it's a very small region -- it's less than one millimeter. And in this small region you have the highest consumption of oxygen in the plants and more important, you have these kinds of signals here. The signals that you are seeing here are action potential, are the same signals that the neurons of my brain, of our brain, use to exchange information. Now we know that a root apex has just a few hundred cells that show this kind of feature, but we know how big the root apparatus is of a small plant, like a plant of rye. We have almost 14 million roots. We have 11 and a half million root apex and a total length of 600 or more kilometers and a very high surface area.

Mancusco speaks as well of plant communication. Not only do they communicate. But it seems they may also be capable of manipulating the behavior of potential pollinators:

Plants are even able to communicate -- they are extraordinary communicators. They communicate with other plants. They are able to distinguish kin and non-kin. They communicate with plants of other species and they communicate with animals by producing chemical volatiles, for example, during the pollination. Now with the pollination, it's a very serious issue for plants, because they move the pollen from one flower to the other, yet they cannot move from one flower to the other. So they need a vector -- and this vector, it's normally an animal... This is a serious business. We have the plants that are giving to the animals a kind of sweet substance -- very energizing -- having in exchange this transportation of the pollen. But some plants are manipulating animals, like in the case of orchids that promise sex and nectar and give in change nothing for the transportation of the pollen.

Those who have explored the healing power of plants through the hallucinogen known as Ayahuasca, speak of the woody vine as "mother Ayahuasca." The experience in an Ayahuasca ceremony led by a Curanero may be experienced as involving a deep connection with the plant as a distinct consciousness. The drink, which is a mixture of the vine and other plants, opens the doors of perception. Is it possible that encoded in the drink's chemistry is a mechanism that switches on communication with the plant and its spirit realm?

A gentler approach to tuning into plant and tree consciousness is through vibrational essences such as produced by us (the authors of these words) that hold the resonance of trees. Our own experience is that opening to the resonance of trees facilitates emotional healing and well being, provides support for us on our spiritual journeys and brings along with it a heightened sensitivity to the plant realm.

Speaking of heightened sensitivity, when the winter of 1998 brought an ice storm - awesomely beautiful yet destructive, that paralyzed central and eastern Canada for more than a week and devastated huge swathes of forest (Under the weight of ice, branches and boles snapped like matchsticks while more flexible trees bent over as if touching their toes) – people were measurably upset by the sight of the broken trees. Everywhere sorrow was expressed. I did not hear anyone openly asking what the trees might be feeling (or whether they might be feeling anything at all), yet I sensed an unvoiced sentiment that the trees were indeed 'experiencing' distress.

Is the feeling that the trees might experience pain the result of a heightened sensitivity, or is it mere human projection or fantasy to think that they might feel, even cry out when they are hurt?

"Wisdom is not knowing
who you are
Only then can you be
Vibrantly unprotected,
Open and accepting
Of all that occurs
What we could learn
from a tree."
—Stuart Schwartz, *The Great Undoing – Dissolving the Me into the Infinite*

Meeting with a Purple Beech

G. and I were walking in a city park in Halifax, Nova Scotia one summer. On this day, whether because we were particularly receptive or for some other reason, the trees seemed to greet us. We felt welcomed, surrounded by wonderful company. G. had just returned from Hamburg, Germany where she had encountered a Purple Beech that had stood for centuries somehow protected from the forces of local history: For her this had been a meeting with a remarkable fellow being. As we continued our walk in the Halifax park we came upon a mature Purple Beech that might have been planted a century ago. G. was at once overcome with feeling and embraced the tree. The moment flooded us with an indescribable warmth and sense of delight. It felt like the tree appreciated this meeting as much as G. or I did.

Connecting with one tree of a certain kind seems to forge a connection with that type of tree no matter where it is found, as if trees of a species form a vast interconnected matrix.

"The apple tree never asks the beech how he shall grow, nor the lion, the horse, how he shall take his prey."
—William Blake, *The Marriage of Heaven and Hell*

Weeping Willows

While researching the possibility of making healing essences from trees that would be especially beneficial for children, G., who was teaching kindergarten at the time spoke with her class about trees. Sure enough, trees we loved as children are also the favorites of her class, Weeping Willow topping the list. So one summer night G., her 8-year old son, Jason, and I set out to the Dominion Arboretum, found in Canada's capital city of Ottawa. There was a line of older Weeping Willows that followed the contours of what is called Dow's Lake. There was a full moon and I planned to make an infusion over this night that would capture the energy imprint from a number of these trees. As I went about my task by the first tree I watched the sun lowering in the eastern sky. A young man was throwing a Frisbee to two dogs, a large Doberman and another tiny breed. The dogs were clearly friends. They both chased after the Frisbee then played tug of war. Jason laughed uproariously at their antics. Nearby two lovers sat on the grass, then eventually got up and walked arm and arm into the setting sun.

It felt like the Weeping Willow had cast its spell, attracting a certain playful energy around it. Undoubtedly, it had its own special qualities, unlike those of any other tree, expressed outwardly in its deeply furrowed bark and wonderfully twisting form. Isn't this outer form and beauty a language, not of words, but something that speaks to us deeply?

"As trees of enchantment, willows formed groves so magical that poets, artists, musicians, priests and priestesses sat within them to gain eloquence, prophecy and inspirational skills through meditation. Because of the willow's close relationship with water, the element pulled into tides by the magnetism of the moon, it has always been considered a feminine tree with a great effect upon the vision-producing subconscious."
—Jacqueline Memory Paterson, *Tree Wisdom*

"Notice that the stiffest tree is most easily cracked, while the bamboo or willow survives by bending with the wind."
—Bruce Lee

"The oak tree is firm and elegant and upright. The weeping willow has allowed the burdens of life to bend it."
—Panache Desai, *Discovering Your Soul Signature: A 33-Day Path to Purpose, Passion & Joy*

Receiving Answers to Questions
Through Asking the Trees

If you ask a tree a question, a true question, sincerely, you may find answers, even seemingly in a magical way. How does that happen? In certain energy of receptivity, we open our psyches and imaginations. Perhaps it is that life each moment is giving us answers... but trees seem to facilitate this process. The best times might be early morning or evening at sunset, times of the full moon when energy is at its peak. Bring a notebook or a recorder. Walk with the trees. Be there and notice. The signs may be all around you. Say, for example, you have questions regarding a child and as you open yourself in the presence of a tree or trees in a place, you notice children playing, laughter or a child climbing a tree. Note this event carefully, attentively, as it may reveal something to you. The answers from trees may come in words or images or in seemingly coincidental events. The great psychiatrist, Carl Gustav Jung, coined a word for this. He called it synchronicity or meaningful coincidence.

If, as the researcher Stefano Mancuso says, the root apex of plants has a tiny portion that serves as a brain and roots act as a sort of neuro network, then perhaps trees have a deep intelligence, different from our own, but capable of helping us find answers to our questions....

So ask a tree and see what signs are revealed!

"In the silence of these groves, we touch reality and see ourselves in clear perspective in relation to our cosmos."
—Richard St. Barbe Baker, *The Redwoods*

"Nature loves to hide. The Lord whose oracle is at Delphi neither speaks nor conceals but gives signs."
—Heraclitus, Greek Philosopher, 5th century B.C.

"If writing novels is like planting a forest, then writing short stories is more like planting a garden. The two processes complement each other, creating a complete landscape that I treasure. The green foliage of the trees casts a pleasant shade over the earth, and the wind rustles the leaves, which are sometimes dyed a brilliant gold. Meanwhile, in the garden, buds appear on the flowers, and colorful petals attract bees and butterflies, reminding us of the subtle transition from one season to the next."
—Haruki Murakami, *Blind Willow, Sleeping Woman*

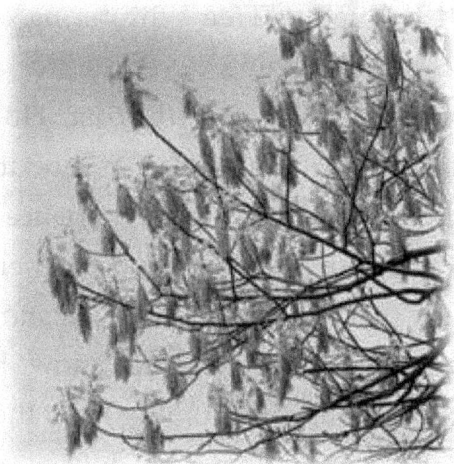

Chapter 19: Tree Whispering

Jim Conroy and Basia Alexander

Dr. Jim Conroy, PhD, The Tree Whisperer®, and Ms. Basia Alexander explain that the word "whisper" as defined in the dictionary means to speak softly and privately with another. "Whispering" with horses, dogs, babies, one's own body, and even microbes became popular in the 1990s. The concept has come to signify an intuitive and deeply felt understanding of—or emotional kinship with—the "other" in ways that conventional science does not advocate or even approach.

With the name "Tree Whispering" you might think that it means leaning close to a tree and saying things very softly. You may do that. However, the main focus of Tree Whispering is about having a deeply personal and profound experience of mutual connection with the Life Force and bioenergy field of a living Being that happens to be green and has leaves and roots. It's about getting to know humanity's partners on the planet and coming from their point of view. Tree Whispering opens the door to cooperating with these Green Beings and forming partnerships with them.

What does it mean to come from anyone's point of view? Perhaps your spouse, child, friend, or a coworker has said, *"Gee, if you could see it through my eyes, then you would understand."* Trees, plants, and all the living Beings of Nature do have their own point of view and people can experience what their lives are like. How can you do that?

A few graduates share their experiences:

Mike, arborist and holistic land care practitioner: "*I remember what Dr. Jim Conroy, The Tree Whisperer said: 'Forget everything. Forget the botany and the physiology that you know. Forget all the learning and just listen to the tree.' To me, forgetting equates to humility. Humility is tough for me because I am proud of what I know. But, I come from the tree's point of view to hear from the tree, not from me. I walk up to trees, but before I touch them. I say, 'I'd like to come inside. I'd like to listen to you. Do I have your permission?' I'll touch the tree with fingertips of both hands, then with my forehead or with my nose. Sometimes I feel electric impulses. I feel the pulses coming to me and then going back into the tree. I just sense what I am feeling about their lives."*

Alexandra, business owner: *"When I was communing with a tree during the workshop, I believe that I briefly saw the tree's chakras. It was a circular rainbow of vibrating luminous color; it was so beautiful! They were very different from human chakras that I see in my healing work with people. So, I have been able to clearly feel trees' emotionality in their lives."*

Linda, business owner: *"This approach works when communicating with any conscious Being—human, animal, insect, disease organisms, plant, or tree. When you have a question about what their lives are like, the best way to receive information is to wonder about the question and let it go. Trust that you will receive what you need. It is, however, important to ask from your heart field and not your ego."*

David, arborist and business owner: *"I've climbed and worked with trees most of my life, but that first evening in the workshop was an amazing expansion of my conscious awareness of trees. I realized that I had always been looking at trees, but not seeing them. I'd always seen*

249

trees move in different ways based on the forces involved or from the way that I would move them as an arborist. But, this was very different. It was Divine in its beauty and its trueness to its growing conditions."

Trees Themselves Describe Their Lives

Blue Spruce in New Jersey: *"We are alive! We are a life form, a Life Force, and valuable assets to humans and all on the planet. We want to be honored for our contribution to humans and as a part of all of Nature. We have a far different form than humans but, like people, have a Life Force that keeps us alive. We are food for the animals and insects; we are home for animals, insects, and organisms. Just as humans want to survive, so do the insects, the animals, and the microorganisms want to survive? We give them a place to do just that."*

Live Oak in California: *"My youth was normal in that I simply thrived here, first as a single trunk, then as a clump, and now "I" am quite merged into a tripod of structures. The trickle of a sweet spring flows up from deep below and nourishes me even in drought. I have maximized my growth to reach for the water as there is ebb and flow from year to year. Thus far, even the most deep of droughts and even the most disruptive of human intrusions nearby have not yet quenched its flow."*

250

Exercise #1: Satellite Views

For another way to come from a tree's point of view and find out what its life is like, try this. Open a mapping engine on your computer. Search for this address: 101 West Montecito Street, Santa Barbara, CA 93101.

Go to the satellite view and zoom in a bit, but not too far. You'll see the famous Moreton Bay Fig tree. You'll also see how roads, parking lots, buildings, and railroad tracks surround it. Imagine living every minute of every day, all year 'round, in this environment. Share the link with a friend, and ask them if they could live that way.

Do an Internet search for other big, historic, important, or champion trees. Put their addresses into a mapping engine and see where and how they live.

"There's a willow tree that stands by my river
She holds me in her arms when I am cold.
And we listen to the sounds
Of the pebbles on the ground,
And I know what it means to be old."
—Douglas Wood

A Shaman's Journey Into the Plant's World

Let's go further, deeper, closer, in, and out. Let's gently set aside our human point of view for a short while and step inside a tree's world.

Cathy, acupuncturist and herbalist: *"I was learning how to meditate while I happened to be sitting next to an old, gnarled Cottonwood. The tree took me inside of it. I went into the center of the trunk. I was on a journey. My consciousness went up and down simultaneously. I heard the vibrations of the leaves. It was like hearing a million tiny violins all playing together, yet I felt that I could hear each one individually. Then, I went into the roots and heard this amazing gong sound. After that, I was inspired to continue meditating."*

By now, you are well prepared for this initiation into mysteries and this sacred journey. Exercises from Chapter 3 of this book prepared you by shifting your mindset into freeing beliefs, expanding sensory perception, establishing trust in your intuition, and learning to come from the other's point of view.

The last bit of advice is this: Don't try to have anyone else's experience. Have your own. Whatever experience comes to you is valid, real, and your personal private interchange with the plant.

What can you expect on this journey? An adventure. You might feel like you are actually moving inside of the plant. You may feel physical sensations like tingling or warmth. You might envision some image in the back of your head or out in front of you. A word or phrase might come into your mind. Some information or insight might occur to you. Happiness, sadness, or any feeling in between might arise within you. A sense of movement, beating, or pulse might come from the plant. Personal memories could also pop up. Thoughts about how the plant operates or how it feels might present themselves to you. The plant may have a clear message for you.

If you think that you are making up those thoughts—you are not. You will know that the thoughts are not yours because you cannot make any certain thought happen. Thoughts simply arrive.

Be trusting and allowing. Maybe you are a bit analytical–not getting into the fun of it. Just remember that this is an adventure. You are stepping into a new world and can bring back a great story to tell.

Are you skeptical? That's okay. There is a place for doubt and questioning as long as you don't let it close your heart to possibilities.

Or, perhaps you hope for so much but you think that nothing is happening! Your expectations put too much stress on you. Just breathe and relax. Start from the top. You can always try it again.

"I wonder if a tree knows when someone's hand is on its body. Does it feel a little warm, like an exchange of electricity? This act of reaching out is a small gesture, but it is filled with great intention. I am simply trying to say hello across the barriers of form and language. I believe the hands communicate this intention most honestly. The voice and mind are not direct enough. Or perhaps they are too complex for the first step of making contact. Besides, the tree and I have such different minds and voices. I don't know the language of alders at all. I can only guess at the shape of a tree's mind and what it knows about life on the edge of a pond. How does this water taste to an alder? How does the morning sun feel on its new leaves? How does the wind feel moving through its branches?"
—Stephanie Kaza, *The Attentive Heart-Conversations with Trees*

Exercise #2: Step Inside a Tree's or Plant's World

Every person going through this exercise will have a different experience. It's best releasing personal judgments, expectations, or agendas.

Read through the steps. Decide whether you feel comfortable doing this exercise. If you do not feel comfortable or have any concern whatsoever, do not do it. If it's easier, you may get the MP3 at PlantKingdomCommunications.com/storeandmore.

Preparation: Make sure you are in a pleasant and private place where you won't be interrupted for 15-20 minutes. Once you begin, if you are uncomfortable, then stop. Don't do anything that is uncomfortable, unpleasant, or painful for you. There will be times during the exercise that you may want to close your eyes, if you are comfortable doing so.

Do this exercise standing or sitting outside privately with a tree. Or, you may be indoors and have a plant near you that you can touch.

Have your notebook/journal handy to write down some notes about your experiences. It's best to make notations immediately in case you don't remember later.

Questions will be asked during the experience. Answer them privately, inside your mind. You may jot notes for answers.

1. Get comfortable. Breathe deeply and gently. Turn your attention to the tree or plant. Never mind its name. Forget anything that you may know about it.

2. Since it is a living Being, always ask permission to make contact. In your Heart, say to the plant or tree, *"I would like to spend some time with you and get to know you. Is that okay?"* It is unlikely, but if you feel disquiet, you may move to another, or stop. Please respect the wisdom of Nature. You may return another time and ask again. But, this time you will probably feel a sense of calm. That means you have permission from it to continue here.

3. Engage your physical senses. Focus your sight on the stem, trunk, leaves, or flowers. Notice the tiniest details. Then, very gently, touch the plant or tree. Feel the textures. Use a soft focus and perceive the whole plant or tree.

4. Focus for a moment on your own body. You may close your eyes. Around your body, notice your heart's bioenergy field. Imagine that your heart's biofield is like the sun—shimmering with light or radiating with energy. Imagine that the field is increasing in size and intensity.

5. Notice or imagine the bioenergy field of the plant or tree. Imagine that its bioenergy field is also expanding.

6. Your heart's biofield now overlaps with the bioenergy field of the plant or tree. In that overlapping area, information is shared and exchanged, sensory experience is stronger, and emotional perception is heightened. With your eyes closed for about a minute, allow yourself to be aware of any new information, experience, or perception in the bioenergy overlapping state.

7. Like a child at play, engage your imagination and close your eyes. Feel as if you shrink or expand to fit the plant or tree's size. Imagine that there is a door on the stem or trunk. You open it. A bright, white light shines on you, and you step inside the stem or trunk.

8. There are thousands of cells all around you. Imagine reaching out with your hands and touching some cell walls. As you look around, you see little streams going up and down all around you. These are circulating plant fluids. Imagine that a tiny boat comes along. Hop in and begin moving upwards with the flow of the fluids. Continue moving upward.

9. You approach a leaf. The boat docks. You float forward into the leaf. Sense light coming through the upper layers of cells.

10. There is a lot of activity: A bubble of carbon dioxide is captured. A bubble of oxygen is released. Sense the heat from foods being produced.

11. Like a child at play, realize that you are inside the leaf. Ask yourself: What do I sense? What do I notice? What do I realize? And what is important to the plant coming from its point of view? Quietly answer those questions inside yourself. You may jot down a few notes.

12. Inside the leaf, photosynthesis is producing sugar molecules, which are food for the plant. Imagine that you shrink down so small you can jump on a sugar molecule. Ride it into the stream. Travel out of the leaf and down the stem or trunk.

13. Imagine that the stream flows beneath the soil and you gently submerge into the root zone. Imagine that the stream is splitting and narrowing. Your molecule stops on the side of the little stream as food. You step off the sugar molecule.

14. Like a child at play, you are inside the roots. Ask yourself: What do I sense? What do I notice? What do I realize? And what is important to the plant or tree coming from its point of view? Quietly answer those questions for yourself or jot down a few notes.

15. Now, feel yourself expand and grow until you fill the whole plant or tree. Sense all the activity — thousands of things happening and interacting. All

these interactions and feedback loops are its Growth Energy. Almost like a pulse or heartbeat, sense the strength and movement of that Growth Energy. Perceive where it is surging. Find out where it might be weak.

16. Ask yourself, *"What is important to the plant coming from its point of view?"* Quietly answer those questions or jot down a few notes.

17. Enjoy a few minutes as if you were being the tree or plant.

18. Now, begin to feel what its life is like in that place. Briefly open your eyes and see where it lives: In sunshine or shade? In open or cramped area? With other trees/plants or alone? With others such as birds, insects, or disease organisms? What is the soil like? Does it have any ropes or ties around it? What is its life like?

19. Be open to receiving a message, image, symbol, or other kind of communication from the tree or plant. Write it down.

20. Feel a two-way flow of connection between you and the tree or plant. Acknowledge that you and the tree or plant have created a conscious partnership. Feel the collaboration between the two of you like a two-way street.

21. Slowly and gently, wiggle your toes and return to your own body and to your own point of view.

22. Realize that you have made a new friend. Realize that your connection allows you to come from the tree's point of view and to know what its life is like.

23. Breathe in any gift from the plant. Breathe out and say *"Thank You"* to the plant for letting you into its world.

24. Please write notes about your experience. If necessary, sit quietly with your pen poised on the paper. Try writing some pleasant words just to get the pen moving.

25. Share your experience with another person who would appreciate it.

"They say that an oak tree is brought into creation by two forces at the same time. Obviously, there is the acorn from which it all begins, the seed which holds all the promise and potential, which grows into a tree. Everybody can see that. But only a few can recognize that there is another force operating here as well-the future tree itself, which wants so badly to exist that it pulls the acorn into being, drawing the seedling forth with longing out of the void, guiding the evolution from nothingness to maturity. In this respect, say the Zens, it is the oak tree that creates the very acorn from which it was born."
—Elizabeth Gilbert, *Eat, Pray, Love*

Asking Questions and Receiving Answers

People often feel that they can control Nature, should dominate the things that they don't like, and are superior because of their scientific knowledge. There is an *imbalance* in the culture and even subtly in our own lives. We human beings often assume that we know best. We usually act based on whatever we want. We often don't ask questions.

We tend to come from the human point of view because we are human. We do this all the time *without even realizing it.* Coming from our own human and personal life's point of view is usually invisible to us, insidious, and might be dangerous to others. Just ask a plant that has been sprayed, pruned, transplanted, or subjected to human folly.

That plant "knows"—not intellectually but at a level of consciousness—that its normal physiology has been insulted if not its life threatened. All living Beings know how to grow, how to live, how to thrive. So, it's best to ask them.

Asking a plant, querying an insect, or talking to a microorganism or any other living Being about its life is the golden opportunity for people to gain intuitive knowing, wisdom, and take actions in collaboration with the other inhabitants of planet Earth. If there is to be a thriving future for humanity on Earth, *Collaboration with Nature* is the mindset in which human behavior must take place.

It's only respectful to ask questions. Asking questions leads to partnership. With a Nature Being such as a tree, plant, insect, bee, microorganism, bird, reptile, deer, or any other, it's like playing the game "20 Questions." When you ask a question, it is posed to the consciousness or spirit of the living Being. For a tree or plant, you may be touching it. But for others, the organism doesn't have to be present. You can make a heart-based and consciousness connection, not a physical connection. Do this especially if you want to converse with an organism that could be dangerous in any way.

In previous exercises you made an intuitive connection and probably received a message from a Green Being. It works in a similar way when you ask specific questions to any Nature Being. Instead of receiving a general message, you ask the kind of question that can be answered with either "yes" or "no" answer. Then you experience that answer in your own sensory systems and intuition.

What Kind of Responses Can You Get?

Clear, "yes" and "no" answers can come through your sensory systems. When you select a signal that works for you, the more you use it the more it is trained into your nervous system.

You can choose to hear the words "yes" and "no" in your inner hearing or select a certain bell sound or tone for each. For the sense of sight, you may decide to see colors such as red for "no" and green for "yes." Or you may select a certain consistent imagery in your mind's eye for each.

For the sense of touch that involves movement, you may choose a specific set of sensations such as gut feelings, a surge of energy that goes up or down, or a set of different tingles. Or as another example, you might shake your head up and down for "yes," then sideways for "no." For the sense of touch that involves knowing at a distance, you may choose a set of knowings that you can relate to.

Receiving signals through the senses of smell or taste is a bit unusual but possible. You may receive certain sets of odors or flavors, each dedicated to a "yes" or "no."

Many people enjoy a combination of senses as signals. You could have a merging of two senses that serve as a single signal. For example, you might hear the word "yes" and see green at the same time.

"As the poet said, 'Only God can make a tree' —probably because it's so hard to figure out how to get the bark on."
—Woody Allen

"Suburbia is where the developer bulldozes out the trees, then names the streets after them."
—Bill Vaughan

"I think that I shall never see
A billboard lovely as a tree.
Perhaps, unless the billboards fall,
I'll never see a tree at all."
—Ogden Nash

What Kind of Questions Should I Ask?

What kind of questions should a person ask to a Nature Being? The best first question is *"May I have your permission to (fill in the blank)."* Asking anyone for permission sets the scene for mutual consideration.

Then, generally, you can ask the same kind of questions you might ask another person: *"Do you want this_____?" "May I do _____for you?" "I want to do _____; does that work for you?"*

More specifically, you might ask these kinds of questions to a tree or plant:

____Do you have sufficient water available? Not enough? Too much?

____Are you connected with the Earth energy?

____Do you have a tie or band that needs to be removed?

____Do you have sufficient nutrients available? If not, would you like organic compost? Would you like it according to the package directions?

____Are you happy with living where you live? Do you want to move to another place? Can you show me where would be best for you? I will point to certain places and ask you whether that is the place you want.

_____Do you need more love or appreciation?

After asking questions, always remember to say "thank you" to the plant for participating in this collaborative encounter. Then, congratulate yourself! You have offered a high level of respect to a fellow passenger on the planetary ship. By offering respect, you have set the foundation for a world that works for everyone. Yes, a simple act—something you would always do with another person—can transform your relationship with the Nature Kingdoms and the whole world.

Could a tree or other living being actually say "no" to a person? They could. By asking a question, you are not imposing your will so the other Being could decline. Given some people's assumption that they are supremely correct and what they want is all that matters, getting a "no" answer from a Nature Being can be startling.

Sometimes, it is not in the best interests of a tree, plant, or other being to receive whatever you are offering to it. So, it will respond "no." However, Nature Beings really, really, want to collaborate with us humans. They know that we are all in this global boat together and it would be better not to sink. So, very often a *"no"* simply means *"ask another, better question"* or *"ask your question another way."* Let a *"no"* response be a guide to lead you to a better way by asking more questions. Be persistent!

"Maybe" answers are possible and often feel ambiguous. Sometimes a long series of "no" answers is the same as a "maybe." Either way, it usually means that you must calm yourself, drink some water or take a break, and begin again with some new questions.

You may get an intuitive idea or a message that will lead you to the right line of further specific questioning.

"You can't sow an apple seed and expect to get an avocado tree. The consequences of your life are sown in what you do and how you behave."
—Tom Shadyac

"Of all the wonders of nature, a tree in summer is perhaps the most remarkable; with the possible exception of a moose singing 'Embraceable You' in spats."
—Woody Allen

Advice for Getting Clear Answers

A tree or plant's Growth Energy or bioenergy field is using your nervous system to provide responses to your questions. Be in that place of inner peace and quiet to allow the overlapping energy fields to exchange information. Honor your intuition and your body's feelings; never do anything that is uncomfortable or painful.

Work fresh. Breathe. Drink Water! If you are tired or thirsty, your answers will be fuzzy. So, slowing down and breathing is very helpful.

Stay neutral, don't impose your will. You might think that you know what an answer should be. Simply note, as an observer, that you have a preference and do your best to release it.

Having doubts? Trust the answers you get! Accept that inner chatter is likely to occur. Don't second-guess your answers; always take the first answer.

Even if your answers don't make logical sense, trust your intuitive responses. Most people have a cultural bias toward left-brain logic to gain answers. Tree Whispering cultivates the practice of accessing right brain and heart-oriented intuitive processes.

Trust comes with practice.

Some people feel nothing but get accurate "yes" and "no" responses.

"Even if I knew that tomorrow the world would go to pieces, I would still plant my apple tree."
—Martin Luther

"One time, when I was very little, I climbed a tree and ate these green, sour apples. My stomach swelled and became hard like a drum, it hurt a lot. Mother said that if I'd just waited for the apples to ripen, I wouldn't have become sick. So now, whenever I really want something, I try to remember what she said about the apples."
—Khaled Hosseini, *The Kite Runner*

"Some of Bay's fondest memories were of lying under the apple tree in the summer while Claire gardened and the apple tree tossed apples at her like a dog trying to coax its owner into playing catch."
—Sarah Addison Allen, *First Frost*

Giving Back to Nature

On your quiet walks in the woods, do you allow yourself to touch or hold a tree? Do you sit with your back leaning on it? When you feel the sense of renewal while walking, do you notice whether the trees are healthy? Do you give anything back to them?

Feeling connected with Nature does not have to be a one-way street. When the human's world and the plant's world overlap, a dynamically balanced cycle of vitality and even an exchange of Spirit become possible. Each helps the other. Just as a tree makes you feel good, you can make a tree healthier. You can give back to trees, plants, and all of Nature's Beings.

"In the cherry blossom's shade
there's no such thing
as a stranger."
—Kobayashi Issa

Exercise #3: Giving Appreciation Followed with Good Practices

One of the processes Dr. Jim Conroy and Basia teach is appreciation of trees and plants. It couldn't be simpler. For at least one minute, say to a tree, plant, or other Nature Being, *"I appreciate your beauty. I am grateful for your life."* Repeating those words becomes like a chant or a hymn. You are drawn deeper and deeper into the truth of it, moving into the shared joy of being alive. Then, follow up with good practices.

1. Pay attention! Look carefully at the greenness and sturdiness of leaves.

2. Check for ties or bands that might strangle and remove them if they are not already totally grown into the bark.

3. See if the plant is pot-bound. Even a tree outside can become pot-bound when it is growing in a very small space. Potted plants can be transplanted or their soil augmented. Give special care to a pot-bound outdoor tree as follows.

4. Soil health is vital. It needs to have living components—microorganisms—in addition to being loose so that roots can push through it. Organic leaf compost is a tree's best friend, preferably made from its own leaves. A very thin layer of shredded leaves all the way out to the drip line keeps roots warm and

soil fertile. Avoid any kind of intrusive practices such as air spading. There are other—organically based—ways to loosen the soil and get more air into it.

5. Do Not "Volcano" Mulch. In other words, don't pile up mulch of any kind around the base of a tree. Roots need air and friendly bacteria—too much mulch can suffocate and kill the bacteria and the tree. One-half to one inch of mulch is plenty. Similarly, Never use fill around a tree, especially during or after construction. Fill Kills.

6. Fertilizing is optional outdoors. Follow label directions for potted plants indoors, and find organic products that have micronutrients. Outside, determine soil fertility by having soil tested by a reputable laboratory. Often, you will find that the soil is adequately fertile. More emphasis on healthy microorganisms in the soil, such as those in organic leaf compost, actually frees-up nutrients in the soil. For a very old tree, it's usually better not to give it any fertilizer until you know it is healthy on the inside by asking it. In human terms, that would be like giving a sexual enhancement drug to a ninety-year-old man without checking his blood pressure.

7. Remember to give the trees water during extremes of drought or heat. A large Oak can transpire 110 to 200 gallons of water a day through its leaves. A week without water in hot summer temperatures is a

drought to any tree. Put a drip hose around the tree at the base and another either at the furthest reaches of the leaves (the "drip-line") or on an uphill slope for a few hours during the night or very early morning. Do this as appropriate to the species depending on heat or dry conditions.

8. Bad pruning can hurt a tree or plant more than not pruning it at all. Research best pruning practices. Find a professional who has rapport and warmth, not only with his or her human customers but also with tree clients.

9. We strongly recommend organic products and approaches. The tree or plant doesn't have a liver like people do. It has to work hard and use precious resources in its internal biochemical "recycling centers" to break down the cocktail of nonorganic constituents in various products. When in doubt about the right organic product, ASK the tree or plant.

10. If you have a backyard or land, start a compost pile. Leaf and kitchen scrap compost or compost teas are excellent organic soil amendments for keeping trees and plants healthy.

Trees, Plants and Others Get Stressed, Too

Which comes first—insects and diseases or weakness in the tree's health? Weakness in the tree's inner health generally calls forth insects and diseases. When a tree is sick, it sends out a signal that attracts them. Many people think that diseases and insects cause weakness in trees and plants. They do, but it is additive. That is, the internal workings of the tree or plant were initially weak, which attracted the insects or diseases. Just like you and me, if we are tired or stressed then we are more susceptible to catching a cold.

Extremes in the environment are the most common stress factors for trees and plants. Here, I mean too hot, too cold, too wet, too dry, or some combination. These are additive over seasons and years. Many people think that when rain finally comes after a hot and dry spell, the trees will absorb water and be fine. Healthy trees might do that. However, to a tree that is already stressed, it may have a blocked circulation system so heat and dryness cause additive damage.

Even with the best of intentions, people sometimes do the wrong things. Trees and plants may be planted in poor soil or in the wrong place. Just like a person, a tree or plant needs to breathe, to drink water, and to live in a clean, bright place.

Stress factors can create a vicious, downward cycle. If a tree or plant is already in poor health or is stressed, another stress factor worsens its physiological health. Three or more stress factors lead to a condition called decline. A single additional stress factor after several stresses usually tips the balance. The tree is trapped; its interior processes can no longer compensate and cannot operate to support the life of the tree.

Disease organisms and insects move in after other stress factors weaken a tree. Most people usually only see the insects and diseases; they focus on the later stages of the whole weakening process. So, believing in a quick fix, people throw on a fertilizer or a pest-killer, hoping that the tree will get better.

There is both ignorance and misinformation about how trees and plants live and maintain their health. But, it doesn't have to be a mystery. Their parts, inner systems, and functions operate much like those of humans. There are many parallels. Functions within the tree or plant need to be addressed in order to truly restore health and vitality.

In modern thinking about tree and plant care, it often goes unrecognized that when a tree gets stressed, its internal functionality becomes compromised. Conventional approaches recommend applying products to the plant or the soil. We say that approach is backwards. Once the timing, rhythm, and balance of bio-interactions within a whole living organism are restored, then I recommend doing the right conventional things to support the activities of new growth.

"Look at the cherry blossoms!
Their color and scent fall with them,
Are gone forever,
Yet mindless
The spring comes again."
—Ikkyu

"If the cherry trees had to wait for understanding they'd never blossom."
—Marty Rubin

Trees, Plants, and Others Can Be Healed

Is it possible to heal a tree's inner health? Can you really heal plants that are sick or in decline? **Yes**! Their inner functionality can be restored to balance and harmony. You can do this easily through bioenergy healing interactions with their biofields in simple, easy ways.

Since products or invasive techniques can't restore inner operability to a tree, what can? Healing Whispers® can. Healing Whispers are focused, intentional, conscious messages or directions conveyed from the heart.

Conscious intentionality works. Research by the Institute of Noetic Sciences into conscious intentionality shows that people; co-create their circumstances and their worlds through their intentionality and conscious interactions with life. Even though physical processes cannot explain consciousness, the use of intentionality and consciousness has a real impact on physical processes.

When offering a Healing Whisper to a nature being, there is a convergence between a person's caring or healing intent and a tree or plant's natural programming to be healthy. Restoration of priority inner operations in a tree or plant occurs in its biofield interactions. There is a re-patterning of its Life Energy or internal processes. This Tree Whispering method of healing trees and plants is similar to successful bioenergy practices used on people including Touch for Health® or The BodyTalk System®. Such human-oriented methodologies attempt to remove blockages and bring inner balance. These techniques are used increasingly in forward-thinking hospitals.

"My nose remembers more than my eyes. The sharp oily smell of eucalyptus combines with afternoon dust from the hockey field. But my heart feels the different then and now."
—Phyllis Theroux, *The Journal Keeper: A Memoir*

"She made me a stranger unto myself, she was all of those calm nights and tall eucalyptus trees, the desert stars, that land and sky, that fog outside..."
—John Fante, *Ask the Dust*

Whispering to Save Trees in a Hurricane

Whispers can save trees; they empower people. Successful use of the Storm Prep Whispers™ helped countless people save their trees before, during, and after Hurricane Sandy on the east coast of the U.S.A. in 2012.

Shelagh W., Mountain Lakes, New Jersey: *"Throughout the storm night, my four children (20, 18, 18, and 13) remained with me. When the winds would really howl, I would say out loud, "Bend trees, bend! Dance with the wind." Initially my kids looked at me as if I had five heads. But, within the hour, they too were shouting over the wind, "Bend trees!! BEND!!" All of my majestic trees stood tall and danced except for one, the tallest, took the hit for the whole community. Your work has profoundly changed my relationship with the trees. Your Whispers helped me prepare physically but more importantly, emotionally for the storm and for the aftermath in my area hit very hard by Hurricane Sandy."*

Ellie C., Hackettstown, New Jersey: *"The day before the storm I went to all of our trees and placed my hands on each one and read the Storm Prep Whispers to them. The storm came and the fierce winds were howling and scary, but I just kept sending my trees love, support,* and confidence. Not one tree fell down even though they seemed to be bending in half. We just had small branches in our yard. I believe it was this work that saved my trees because our neighbors lost two 60-foot evergreens."

Alison, Randolph, New Jersey: "*Our trees were well prepared with the Storm Prep Whispers and made it through the storm really well. We didn't lose any trees at all, although our neighbors lost several big ones. We only lost a few smaller branches.*"

Christina K., Bergen County, New Jersey, "*I spoke to all of the trees surrounding my property with the Storm Prep Whispers. I could feel the trees sending their roots deeper and all of them dropped their leaves—all except for one. This big Maple in my neighbor's yard still had green and yellow leaves. I spoke to him again. He replied "Don't worry, I've got this!" I told him he didn't have to do it the hard way; he could drop his leaves so that the winds wouldn't hurt him. The next day the leaves facing my house turned brown and dropped. But, three-quarters of the rest of the tree still had green and yellow leaves!! It was as if he did this just for me! After the storm, there was no damage—no limbs came down at all. Yet a block away, a huge tree fell, bringing down power lines and pulling up the sidewalk. That gives you an idea of how bad the winds were here.*" Please read more stories in our book *People Saving Their Trees In Hurricane Sandy.*

Exercise #4 Become A Tree Healer with the Healing Whispers

When you do the Healing Whispers, you are addressing the wisdom or consciousness of all of Nature to help with your intentional requests. That is why the Whispers are said with the word *"please."*

Read through the steps. Decide whether you feel comfortable doing this exercise. If you do not feel comfortable or have any concern whatsoever, do not do it.

Preparation: Do this exercise outside either privately with a tree or while you take a walk in the woods. Or, you may do the Healing Whispers indoors with potted plants.

1. Breathe gently and feel connected with Nature.

2. In your mind and heart, say these Healing Whispers one to five times to a single sick tree or keep repeating them to all of Nature's living Beings as you walk.

3. Please release blockages and distribute growth energy where it is needed.

4. Please orchestrate inner parts, feedback loop systems, and functions to play in harmony.

5. Please connect all ecosystem members' Life Force and bioenergy fields into community and balance

each with the other (including "invasives" and people), in peace.

6. I love these Beings and collaborate with them so al survive and thrive.

7. When you feel complete, you may ask for any messages from the trees or other Nature Beings. Be sure to write their messages down.

8. Say *"thank you."* And take a moment to write some notes about your experience.

9. Make a plan to return and repeat this Healing Whispers process.

You may go to TreeWhispering.com/Whispers to request a free postcard-size version of these Healing Whispers.

"Late in August the lure of the mountains becomes irresistible. Seared by the everlasting sunfire, I want to see running water again, embrace a pine tree, cut my initials in the bark of an aspen, get bit by a mosquito, see a mountain bluebird, find a big blue columbine, get lost in the firs, hike above timberline, sunbathe on snow and eat some ice, climb the rocks and stand in the wind at the top of the world on the peak of Tukuhnikivats."
—Edward Abbey, *Desert Solitaire*

Mutual Healing

When people help trees and plants regain health with the techniques of Tree Whispering, the people usually feel good, too. Unselfish concern, kindness, courage, and compassion offered to others are heart-based emotions which HeartMath Institute research shows are physically and emotionally beneficial to the person offering them.

While doing the Healing Whispers, your own heartbeat was probably slow and regular, chemicals associated with good feelings may have entered your bloodstream, your breathing was likely to be regular and deep, and your emotional state was probably calm, peaceful, or even inspired. So there may have already been a kind of mutual healing occurring just by doing the exercises of this chapter and offering Healing Whispers to the Beings of Nature.

Alan, PhD psychologist: *"When I was in graduate school, there was little credence given to the mind-body connection. But, things have changed. Now we know that giving up focus on self and opening the heart in communication with other Beings results in benefits for a person that can be measured as reduced inflammation, less anxiety, and less distress. So it works both ways: by helping trees I feel like they are helping me. For example, Wild Rose taught me to relax and release tension in myself as I pruned it. As long as I was open to it and calm, the wild rose allowed me to trim with my clippers. I worked a branch at a time, often standing in the middle of sprays of canes with big thorns. I didn't get cut. I learned to work with it. It enhanced my patience. I am very fortunate to be in a position where I can spend time with trees, feel their strength and beauty, and communicate with them."*

"If I stand here, I can see the Little Red Haired girl when she comes out of her house... Of course, if she sees me peeking around this tree, she'll think I'm the dumbest person in the world... But if I don't peek around the tree, I'll never see her... Which means I probably AM the dumbest person in the world ... which explains why I'm standing in a batch of poison oak."
—Charles M. Schulz

"... Bookstore, which smelled the way only a new book from England does when you open it for the first time, faintly like nutmeg, dry, erudite."
—Frederick Beuchner

Dr. Jim's Story

I recently experienced a health crisis. In addition to receiving both conventional medical and complementary health treatments, I believe that I receive a kind of healing from trees, plants, and ecosystem members while I heal them. During my health crisis, I received both comforting messages as well as gentle bioenergy scanning. Usually that feeling of 'scanning' gets to a problem spot and stops. It feels like the tree is sending healing energy to that area, and then the 'scan' moves on. So, if I spend an hour using my Tree Whispering and Cooperative BioBalance® systems to treat a tree, I feel as if it is also scanning me for that same hour and sending its healing energy wherever I need it.

About a year ago, I was having problems with my kidneys. I went to a Beech tree that was over one hundred years old. It had a couple of small bleeding phytophthora spots on it. When I started to treat the tree by using my conscious intentionality and with bioenergy fields overlapping, I heard the tree say, *"If you help me with my spots, I will help you with your spots."* In other words, by helping the tree become healthier and its disease spots clear, the tree would help my kidney problems clear. Sure enough, one year later, we were both clear!

I was also having a urinary system problem at the same time. I went to a big old Oak tree that was having circulation problems. The Oak tree said, "If you help me open up my tubes [xylem and phloem], I'll help you open up your tubes [urinary tract]. I have since had surgery on my urinary system. The surgery was successful even though I was given only a 50/50 chance of success.

Trees and plants are naturally the most generous of Beings. Tree Whispering students tell us stories about feeling that they were receiving healing energies from trees or plants that were themselves quite sick. Nature Beings really want to help humans.

We must, however, re-issue this warning. When doing any of these exercises with trees, plants or any Nature Being, you should be receiving positive information and pleasant sensations, not pain or discomfort of any kind. If you feel pain inside your body or psychological discomfort, stop the exercise immediately. Develop strong, healthy personal and psychological boundaries before you connect with and work with a tree, plant, or any Nature Being. Use good, common sense to take care of yourself.

Exercise #5 Mutual Healing with a Nature Being

Mutual healing, as the phrase implies, is a two way street: It's giving *and* receiving. So offering the Healing Whispers is a vital part of the upcoming exercise. It's polite to offer a healing-type action to another before requesting something in return. Also, the tree or plant involved needs to be in a healthier state in order to offer you some of its Life Force. Also, when you review the Healing Whispers, you can imagine that those directives could generally apply to human bodies and their inner ecosystems as well.

You know that we have to remind you of these important points:

If you feel that you are sick in some way or have some kind of health crisis, you must seek medical advice and/or treatment. Do not use this exercise as a substitute.

If you feel that you would benefit from a shared experience with a Nature Being, please approach doing this exercise out of curiosity and in the spirit of fun.

Set your expectations in a realistic way: Do not expect that this exercise alone will heal you of any condition or crisis. You may expect to have a neutral, or generally positive, or generally beneficial experience.

The authors and publishers are not responsible for your well being in any way. You are responsible for your own well being. Take authority for your own life. Use good common sense about taking care of yourself. Don't do anything that is uncomfortable.

Recall in chapter 3, exercise #6, you were asked to breathe and gently tap on both side of your head and on your heart area. Gentle tapping is a proven technique for stimulating the body—particularly the Chinese healing system of meridian points—so that the nervous system and other systems are operating in sync. We'll use breathing and tapping in this exercise, too. If you are standing or sitting with a single tree or plant, please gentle tap on its trunk or stem initially. Then, if you can easily reach, you may tap on the soil area where the roots are at the base of the trunk or stem. If you are walking, don't bother doing the tapping.

Read through the steps of this exercise. Decide whether you feel comfortable doing this exercise. If you do not feel comfortable or have any concern whatsoever, do not do it.

Preparation: Do this exercise outside privately with a tree or indoors with potted plants in a place where you won't be interrupted for about 15 to 20 minutes.

1. Breathe gently and feel connected with Nature as you have done in previous exercises. Have the feeling of appreciation. As in previous exercises, experience your own heart's bioenergy field glowing and expanding like the sun. Be aware that the tree or plant has a bioenergy field. The bioenergy fields expand and overlap. In that overlapping area, information can be exchanged and sensory perception may be stronger.

2. Come from the tree or plants' point of view as best you can. Focus your attention and consciousness on the tree or plants.

3. Ask the tree or plants, *"Do I have permission to engage in this mutual healing exercise with you?"* Receive your *"yes"* or *"no"* signal. If *"no,"* then stop. Please respect the wisdom of Nature. You may return another time and ask again. If *"yes,"* continue here.

4. As in the previous exercise, you may take a moment to ask some yes/no questions about the tree or plants' health. You may focus your attention on various ecosystem members and possibly receive messages from them, too.

5. Think about your own health goal. How do you want to feel? Convey that to the tree or plants.

6. Realize that at the same time as you offer the following Healing Whispers to the tree or plants, it/they may be offering their own kind of "bioenergy scanning" or energy assistance to you.

7. In your mind and heart, slowly say each of these sentences thinking of the tree/plants well being and your health goal at the same time. Gently tap on the trunk or stem as you repeat these sentences. (If it is convenient, you may also tap on the soil area at the base of the tree or plant.)

8. Please RELEASE blockages and distribute Growth Energy where it is needed.

9. Please ORCHESTRATE inner parts, feedback loop systems, and functions to play in harmony.

10. Please CONNECT all ecosystem members' Life Force and bioenergy fields into community and BALANCE all—each with the other (including "invasives" and people) in peace.

11. Pause and open yourself to receive any messages, impressions, or encouragement from the tree or plants. Be sure to write it down.

12. Repeat Steps 7-11 two more times. During those repeats, you may touch the tree or plant with one hand and tap on your own heart area with the other hand. During those repeats, you may touch the tree or plant with one hand and alternate tapping on your own heart area and head with the other hand.

13. When you feel complete, say, *"I love myself and these Beings. I collaborate so that all ecosystem members — including me — may survive and thrive."*

14. Pause and focus on your whole experience. Make notes.

15. Say *"thank you"* and make an arrangement with the tree or plants to return and repeat this process if you would like to do so. Write the "date" into your calendar.

"The nutcracker sits under the holiday tree, a guardian of childhood stories. Feed him walnuts and he will crack open a tale..."
—Vera Nazarian, *The Perpetual Calendar of Inspiration*

"A thing which I regret, and which I will try to remedy some time, is that I have never in my life planted a walnut. Nobody does plant them nowadays — when you see a walnut it is almost invariably an old tree. If you plant a walnut you are planting it for your grandchildren."
—George Orwell

Transformation into a New World

As the 17th Century "Cartesian" worldview developed, people came to believe that they could control Nature, that they should dominate Nature for their own benefits, and that science—as it was being created in the 17th Century—made people superior to Nature.

By the 20th Century, using such a context for thinking—the mindset of control, domination, and superiority—didn't seem to be working out very well for ecological health, cultural stability, or peacefulness among peoples. But now, broader—even universal—truths are surfacing within humanity's consciousness.

Humanity—each and every one of us—is going through something like a computer operating system upgrade. People are realizing that they need to think-outside-of-the-boxes they are accustomed to using. To solve the problems created by those old worldviews, it's not just cleverness, creativity, or technology that will save the day, although all those are needed. Adopting a new mindset and then taking new kinds of actions within that new mindset will make all the difference.

People will have to shift from believing that *"the world is mine for the taking"* to believing *"we are all in this together"* and *"everybody is connected to everybody."* When you and just 10% of the population accept that *Collaboration with Nature* is possible, all people can begin to take actions with Nature Beings out of kindness, compassion, a desire to help, mindfulness, and equality. All may learn to come from the other Being's point of view.

That will be a moment like few others in history. Philosopher and writer of the 19th Century, Victor Hugo, called such powerful junctures in time *"an idea whose time has come"* and added that there is no army stronger. When a new idea sweeps through humanity's consciousness, everything changes. It is like the tide coming in—all boats rise.

"Happiness is free, Mama says, as sure as the blinkin' stars, the withered arms the trees throw down for our fires, the waterproofin' on our skin, and the tongues of wind curlin' the walnut leaves before slidin' down our ears."
—Emily Murdoch, *If You Find Me*

Making the U-Turn from Despair to Empowerment

But, I can imagine you may be thinking: *"It'll never happen." "Things are too bad." "What I do won't make any difference." "It's too late."* ... just to name a few. Some people have a sense of despair for the environment.

But those are just thoughts. No one knows if any of those thoughts, often said in hopelessness, are true. Those are not the final cries of the end. I believe such expressions are the *first* signs of true transformation! All you need is a nudge toward making a u-turn away from feeling hopeless or helpless to set yourself on the path toward making the first small differences which will grow into large differences.

How do you become empowered or enabled to make a difference? First, look at how far you have come. You have already begun by expanding your level of respect for trees and plants as living Beings of Nature. You have begun the shift of your worldview to that of *Collaboration with Nature.* You started to expand your perceptive skills, intuition, and sensory awareness. Then, you practiced coming from the tree or plant's point of view.

Next, turning your own backyard or nearby public park into an island of balance is one of the greatest contributions you can make. You probably already walk the talk of *sustainability* by doing things like recycling and lowering your carbon footprint. By walking the talk of *collaboration* with the Green Beings and other ecosystem members right in your home, your yard, or nearby in Nature, you will be co-creating a world that you would actually want to live in. I call that your *"wanted world."*

Never mind that you think your backyard is a small space. Don't underestimate the power of a small zone of dynamic balance because it spreads throughout the web of life. Balance is more stable than imbalance. With the new paradigm of thought—*Collaboration with Nature*—on your side, you have the power of balance. All you have to do is use the skills you have learned here in daily life.

"Water that never moves," I say to him. "It's fine for a little while. You can drink from it and it'll sustain you. But if it sits too long it goes bad. It grows stale. It becomes toxic." I shake my head. "I need waves. I need waterfalls. I want rushing currents."
—Tahereh Mafi, *Ignite Me (Shatter Me, #3)*

Exercise #6 Thinking At a Higher Level about Nature

I appreciate Albert Einstein's words, *"The significant problems we face cannot be solved at the same level of thinking we were using when we created them."* Instead of reaching back into the prevailing cultural mindset to attempt to solve ecological imbalance, Dr. Jim and I suggest trying on some new ideas about Nature.

Preparation: Read through the points below. Evaluate them for yourself. Are they attitudes or beliefs that you would like to adopt? Like a new shirt, try on one or more of the following new beliefs about Nature.

Do they—or could they—feel true? If so, "buy" the shirt by adopting the belief for yourself. Do any feel tight? Are they the wrong color? Exchange them for something new that fits better. Never do anything that is uncomfortable for you.

Try making posts or tweets out of these new beliefs, too!

1. There is Intelligence in Nature's living Beings. I can communicate with them by using my sensory system and intuition.

2. I listen to my friends in Nature with an open heart. I am their partner.

3. I don't impose my will, I ask Nature what it needs and wants.

4. I come from the plant's point of view; I see how it lives its life.

5. I am an equal part of a greater Whole.

6. Every living Being has a purpose–even "weeds."

7. My personal experience is as valid as any scientific finding.

8. I can heal trees and ecosystems, and that is healthy and healing for me, too.

9. Everybody can win. Everyone-plants, trees, ecosystems-lives through collaboration.

10. Cooperation with the other living Beings of Nature works for me and for them.

11. Collaboration is the new picture-frame through which I see my world.

12. I no longer suffer resignation. I am empowered-can make a difference with the living Beings of Nature in my ecosystems and in my world.

13. I can form partnerships that enhance trees' and plants' ability to survive, with no downside to me. I can live and let others live.

15. A condition of peaceful co-existence can flourish in Nature, permitting health and growth for all, including me. Nobody needs to be killed.

16. Healthy trees, plants, and even "invasives" can co-exist in dynamic balance.

17. Collaborating with Nature is an idea whose time has come.

"Whole forests of oak, beech, poplar, maple, and walnut, standing since Columbus, collapsed ... from girdling and deadening with fire. There was in the heart of the new race no more consideration for the trees than for the game until the best of both were gone; steel conquered the West but chilled the soul of the conqueror. This assault on nature, than which few more frightful spectacles could be imagined, owed much to sheer need, but something also to a compelling desire to destroy conspicuous specimens of the fauna and flora of the wilderness. The origin of this mad destructiveness may be in doubt, but there is no question about its effect. The Ohio Valley today has neither trees nor animals to recall adequately the splendor of the garden of the Indian which the white man found and used so profligately."

—Stephen E. Ambrose, *Crazy Horse and Custer: The Parallel Lives of Two American Warriors*

Live-And-Let-Live and EcoPeace Treaties

A related idea in the *Collaboration with Nature* worldview is *Live-And-Let-Live*. Killing unwanted insects, disease organisms, or other living Beings in an ecosystem has been a common practice. So common, in fact, that the practice has not been questioned. The worn-out framework-of-thought suggests that killing unwanted or "invasive" Beings of Nature is acceptable. Sometimes, killing seems to work temporarily—from the human point of view—but it always disrupts and imbalances the ecosystem. How? By killing off a given population, their absence allows a new population of other organisms—whether they are wanted organisms or not—to have an advantage.

Once ecosystems are healthy, connected, and communicating, then it is possible to work out agreements at the level of consciousness between all the ecosystem members, including "invasives." All ecosystem members–including "invasives"–can live in a state of dynamic balance. A leading edge approach that Dr. Jim Conroy has developed—called EcoPeace Treaties®—is showing that killing is obsolete.

Dr. Jim and Nature's living Beings have devised a way to collaborate without any living being ever having to settle for something less than what is needed to survive. Nobody wins or loses in an EcoPeace Treaty. Everyone is included. Everyone gives, sometimes with generosity. Everyone lives.

Lodgepole Pine trees in Colorado: *"When our fluids are pulsing and we are making food for ourselves, we are growing. Growing is what we want to do; it is what we need to do. To grow, so many things must happen inside of us in the right order and in perfect timing. This is like making music with many instruments. We are healthy on the inside when our song is strong. Then, we can live together with some insect Beings and some disease Beings. All can co-exist."*

An EcoPeace Treaty is always a 3-part structure that is shown visually as an up-side-down triangle. Two organisms that are usually at odds with each other—such as Emerald Ash Borer and Ash trees, bleeding canker disease and Beech or Oak trees, and many others—are placed at the flat top of the triangle. These are the organisms that are considered equals and need to resume mutual communication to come into dynamic balance with each other. The people responsible for the property are represented at the bottom point of the triangle.

The facilitator of the EcoPeace Treaty—usually Dr. Jim Conroy, but it could be you—provide a forum of consciousness in which the Life Force of the living beings can have a meeting. They first express exactly what they need in order to survive and thrive. Then, they collaborate amongst themselves how they can co-exist. Some natural attrition may occur but one organism does not have to wipe out the other organism, and they know that. The facilitator may offer ideas into the forum of consciousness that the living Being may weigh, but *never* attempts to force an outcome on the living Beings. (Forcing wouldn't work anyway. Permission is always required.) The facilitator may represent or may be the property owner. As the third party of the triangle, people need to support the organisms' agreement by doing things such as not killing, not using chemicals, providing good habitat, etc.

Assumed within the EcoPeace Treaty 3-part structure is the human experience of identifying with or experiencing the way life is lived for the organisms–plants, insects, diseases, or any others. EcoPeace Treaties empower people to collaborate by helping Nature's living organisms return to dynamic balance. Thereby, people help themselves live sustainably.

Exercise #7: Forward FROM the Future into Your Wanted World

Going forward FROM the future is like making flight and hotel reservations for a vacation. You know that vacation is some time in the future. But, making the reservations puts a commitment into the timeline. Every action taken from that point forward is taken within the scope of the commitment to take that flight, to stay at that hotel, and to have a wonderful time on that vacation. Does that sound familiar?

We all go forward FROM the future. Our choices, dreams, and intentions are the metaphorical flight-and-hotel-reservations we all make for our lives and for the world.

I (Basia Alexander) have a small notebook. In it, I write descriptions of my wanted world--the world I want to live in. Please let me share some of my ideas with you.

1. In my wanted world, landscapers would ask the consciousness of the trees and plants how they want to live before they (the landscapers) do anything.

2. I live in a world where my apparently small actions to help trees and plants ripple out to become BIG WAVES.

3. I live in a world where builders are sensitive to making changes on the earth and homeowners care

about their trees at least as much as their houses, and will do anything to protect their trees.

4. In my wanted world, nature communication is common; people think it's strange not to ask a tree about its life. They teach their children that invisible beings ARE really there to help Nature grow.

5. I live in a world where everyone—including businesses and governments—has come to their senses and realized that we are all in this together.

6. In my wanted world, the people at the helms of educational institutions have recognized that we are all in this together, and have begun to offer more enlightened, comprehensive, and open-minded courses about personal spirituality, holistic health, and collaboration with nature. The ideas are really becoming popular now!

7. In my wanted world, all living organisms are respected as fellow passengers on Earth/Gaia. People form conscious partnerships with Nature Beings, recognizing that there are no "bad guys." The predominant philosophy is Live-and-Let-Live.

8. In the world I live in, killing is obsolete. Human ingenuity and Nature's wisdom working together make it possible for all to survive and thrive.

9. In my wanted world—and thanks to actions others and I have taken—trees, plants, and ecosystems are balanced to climate extremes and can

thrive despite those changes. In fact, their robust growth is starting to help reverse climate changes.

10. In my wanted world, I have been able to communicate my personal and ecological visions with kindness and courage. My family, friends, and community are starting to accept that the world I want to live in is possible.

I hope the ideas for my wanted world inspire ideas for you. In the musings of a daydream or written on paper, please begin to create the feelings, vision, and perspectives—make your flight and hotel reservations—for the kind of world you would actually WANT to live in.

For the time being, pay less attention to the one you do live in; begin to detail the large and small aspects of the world you want.

Live FROM that future. And so, you will create your wanted future.

"Words are like birds, passing through the trackless sky. The dog barking, the sound of the purling stream, the wind among the weeping willow trees: how are these not right off the tongue of the Buddha?"
--Lama Surya Das, *Awakening To The Sacred: Creating a Spiritual Life from Scratch*

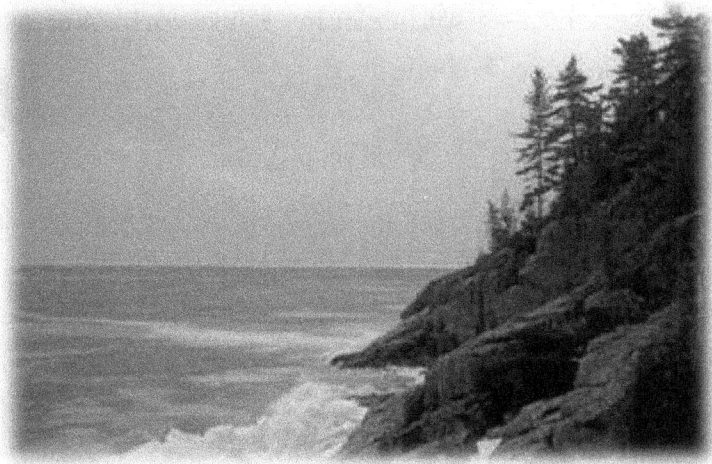

Chapter 20: Creativity and Trees

Daniel Tigner (Hafiz)

Creativity is a potential avenue of healing ourselves and healing our world. When we create we may bring forth and manifest the best in us. The whole creative process can be one of love, integration, discovery, expansion, and wonder with many "Ah Ha," moments! What more delightful subject to engage with then a tree, as expressed in the famous poem of Joyce Kilmer, who died a few years later while serving as a soldier in the First World War, but his simple poem has endured.

"Earth teach me to forget myself as melted snow forgets its life. Earth teach me resignation as the leaves which die in the fall. Earth teach me courage as the tree which stands all alone. Earth teach me regeneration as the seed which rises in the spring."
—William Alexander

"Life will break you. Nobody can protect you from that, and living alone won't either, for solitude will also break you with its yearning. You have to love. You have to feel. It is the reason you are here on earth. You are here to risk your heart. You are here to be swallowed up. And when it happens that you are broken, or betrayed, or left, or hurt, or death brushes near, let yourself sit by an apple tree and listen to the apples falling all around you in heaps, wasting their sweetness. Tell yourself you tasted as many as you could."
—Louise Erdrich, *The Painted Drum*

Trees by Joyce Kilmer (1913)

I think that I shall never see
A poem lovely as a tree.

A tree whose hungry mouth is pressed
Against the earth's sweet flowing breast;

A tree that looks at God all day,
And lifts her leafy arms to pray;

A tree that may in Summer wear
A nest of robins in her hair;

Upon whose bosom snow has lain;
Who intimately lives with rain.

Poems are made by fools like me,
But only God can make a tree.

Getting to Know Trees through Drawing and Painting

When drawing and painting, sculpting, even creating a mosaic – what more beautiful thing to represent than a tree.

Visual arts require astute observation.

When we survey paintings during different periods over the centuries, it is fascinating to see how our perceptions of trees have changed. Once upon a time – go back to the renaissance - trees were stuck in paintings as more or less decoration. Later they became more intricate parts of the landscape. But it was only in the 18th century that artists began to see trees as worthy of being the subject in their own right of their paintings.

Portraying a tree is facilitated, just as in successfully drawing the human figure, by knowledge and a feel for its anatomy. When you really see and feel a tree, understand its birth and growth cycles, how it has experienced the seasons, formed through the elements and the challenges of the environment, then expressing its beauty and power comes more naturally.

It is worthwhile to visit museums to see the great artists. We can learn much from them about seeing trees. And, if we draw or paint, understanding their approach and absorbing their deep involvement can enhance our own efforts at portraying a tree. Here's a simple line drawing on paper of a Ponderosa Pine from Grant Tigner, a wonderful draughtsman. See how the essence of the tree is expressed, not with complex minute details, but simply and economically. Trees as subjects of art invite us to simultaneously express our creative vision while attuning to their presence.

"It is curious how one's feelings about trees change, in proportion to one's appreciation of their importance and dignity as live beings. Trees are individual beings: they can be comic, heroic, tragic to the sensitive, practiced eye of the landscape artist."
—John F. Carlson, *Carlson's Guide to Landscape Painting*

"Life without love is like a tree without blossoms or fruit."
—Khalil Gibran

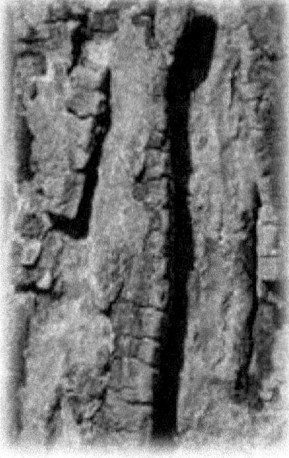

Chapter 21: The Fractal Patterns of the Diversity Tree

Kimberly Burnham

Just noticing the pattern, the way in which we are similar and are connected can bring healing, strengthen the function of your brain, helps you to be more adaptable. This all makes breakfast more fun in the morning, explains Kimberly Burnham.

Many of the patterns in the natural world are fractal in nature. Fractals are a mathematical description of a rough, uneven shape. An oak tree has a fractal shape with a self similar branching pattern.

One of the characteristics of fractal patterns is that the big thing is like the small thing only bigger. A tree for example has a trunk with branches. Each branch with its own branches is like the trunk only smaller. Even tiny leaves have trunk-like veins which branch. The vein in the leaf is like the tree trunk only much, much smaller.

Often your eyes relax when you notice this natural pattern and the similarity of shapes, whether it is a bright red maple tree in the fall or a tall blue spruce or an oak tree seedling. And when we are relaxed, our blood flows through our fractal branching blood vessels bringing nourishing oxygen and nutrients to our fractal patterned brain. There is scientific research that suggests we heal faster and have less pain in a hospital room with windows that looks out over a natural scene with fractal shaped poplar trees, red tulips, blades of blue green grass with fractal shaped mountain ranges, puffy white clouds or a jagged shoreline in the distance.

Try this *Fractal Tree Vision* exercise outside in a place that has trees, when you have a chance. Or you can at each step close your eyes and do this as visualization—imagining a huge beautiful tree that you are familiar with. The healing properties of noticing the natural patterns seems to work even

311

when you are looking at a painting of a tree or natural landscape.

1. Look around yourself. Notice the light. How bright is it? Notice the colors and shapes around you. This is the "before" measurement of how you feel in your own skin and in your environment. Notice how you feel. How relaxed are your head and shoulders. Feel whether every part of your body is comfortable. Take a minute or two to check in with your body and emotions. Then take a minute or two with each of these steps.

2. Choose a tree for this exercises (real or imagined or a painting). Stand about 20 feet or seven meters from the tree. Notice the overall shape. Do you recognize the kind of tree it is? It doesn't matter if you do. Are there any birds that you see or hear? Are there any crickets or bugs making sounds? Is there a wind blowing, moving the tree? Notice the overall color of the leaves and branches.

3. Walk a little closer, so that you are about 10 feet or three meters from the tree. What is different from this distance? Do you notice more detail in the roughness of the bark? Notice the angle at which the branches come off the central trunk. See how the leaves are not all the same color and that there are shades and variation in the leaves. Does your body

312

feel different as you look at the tree from this distance?

4. Now go even closer so that you are about three feet or one meter from the tree. Is there anything new that you notice? Look at the detail in the textures, the edges, how one branch flows into another or how the color on one part of the leaf gradually changes hue. How do your eyes feel now about a meter from the tree?

5. Again even closer so your face is just a few centimeters or inches from the tree. Look at the ridges and swirls in the bark. Is the bark on the trunk different from the bark on the branches or is it a smaller version? Notice the texture of a leaf. Trace the edge with your fingers. Feel the bumpiness.

6. Then close your eyes and imagine you are looking through a microscope at the bark or leaf or fruit or blossom of the tree. What details do you notice? How does the tree feel different to you? How do you feel different?

7. Now reverse the process and back up so you are about three feet or one meter from the tree. What is different from when you were earlier this distance from the tree? Do you notice anything new? Is there a new smell in the air? What has changed?

8. Back up even farther, so you are about 10 feet or three meters from the tree. Do you get a different

feeling from the tree? Does the energy around the tree or around you feel different? Calmer? More charged? What feels different?

9. Now back to the starting place about 20 feet or seven meters from the tree. Take a good look and notice the details, the variation in the shapes and colors of this individual tree.

10. Finally, look around yourself. Notice the light. How bright is it? Notice the colors and shapes around you. This is the "after" measurement. Notice where in your body you feel better. How relaxed are your head and shoulders. See whether every part of your body feels comfortable. Take a minute or two to check in with your physical self and your surroundings.

You have just experienced an individual tree, which is unique and yet has a pattern with the various parts of the tree—a smaller or bigger version of each other.

"Nature's patterns sometimes reflect two intertwined features: fundamental physical laws and environmental influences. It's nature's version of nature versus nurture."
—Brian Greene

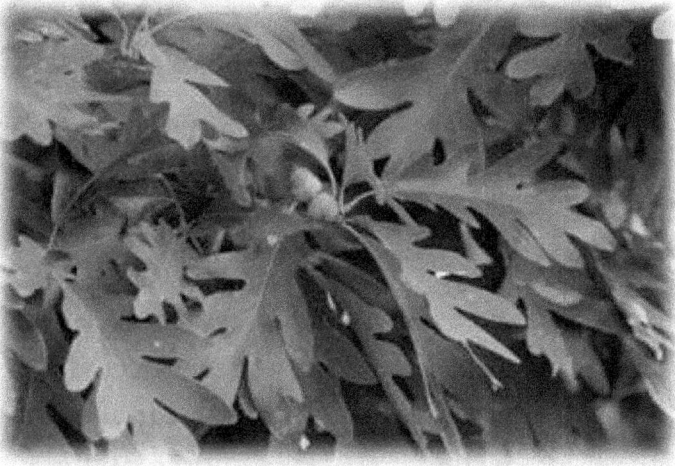

Chapter 22: Photography as a Tool to Train Our Eyes to See Beauty and Patterns in Nature

Daniel Tigner (Hafiz)

A simple phone camera is all one needs to begin tree photography, which is delightful and rewarding for the results we can achieve for trees are majestic and awe inspiring, beautiful, intricate marvels of natural design, says Daniel Tigner (Hafiz). How can we learn to photograph them? What is the key to successfully creating powerful and healing images.

The first thing is to spend time just looking. Look at the trees. See their shape, colors, textures, structures, strengths and weaknesses, what you feel are their lines of energy, how their roots anchor the tree and spread outward and downward. Look at them simply with an appreciative eye, see their qualities, their auras, their grace. Look at them for a few minutes or more every time you get a chance.

A camera is an extension of our eyes. Two people photographing the same thing, at the same time and with the same type of camera will often produce dramatically different results. Through photography we can really see how we see the world. The images we create photographing a tree mirror how we look at the environment. Observe the beauty and grace of a tree, look with loving eyes and you will discover that you begin to see animals and people with a more loving and tender gaze as well - you will convey some quality of healing and kindness.

From a technical point of view photographing trees is both challenging and fun. A wide angle lens is ideal to take a picture of the whole form of a tree, a macro or close up lens helps us capture the details of a flower or a leaf, and a telephoto lens allows us to capture something further away such as a bird's nest in the bough of a tree.

Each lighting situation presents technical challenges as well as aesthetic possibilities. For example, leaves backlit by the sun with their veins and colors brought out can make a wonderful image. On a rainy day the droplets of water on the flowers offer endless possibilities for poetic expression, mixed with the extra technical challenge of working in a darker light.

Make a portrait of a tree, something beautiful and healing! Getting out there and taking pictures is a great way to get to know a tree.

"To control the breathing is to control the mind. With different patterns of breathing, you can fall in love, you can hate someone, you can feel the whole spectrum of feelings just by changing your breathing."
—Marina Abramovic

"The future is there... looking back at us. Trying to make sense of the fiction we will have become."
—William Gibson, *Pattern Recognition*

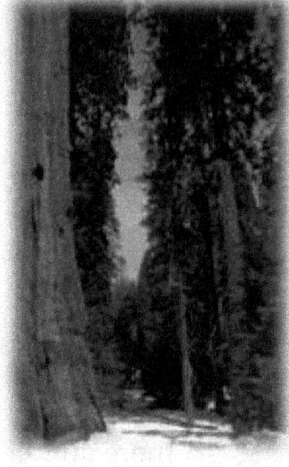

Chapter 23: Music of the Trees

Daniel Tigner (Hafiz)

For almost every musician, trees have been a part of their music simply because so many instruments are made of wood – piano, guitar, recorder, oboe, violin, explains Daniel (Hafiz) Tigner Musician and music lovers, have explored the connection with trees and written music to try to capture the feeling of trees and forest. But a new realm is opening up with the possibility of actually hearing the music of the trees.

Bartholomäus Traubeck has created equipment to try to translate tree rings into records and play them on a turntable. The results are a new class of music.

http://www.iflscience.com/plants-and-animals/what-do-tree-rings-sound-when-played-record

Other researchers are attaching electrodes to plants and translating those signals into sound. North of Piedmont, Italy, researchers from the Damanhur community have been exploring just that since the 1970s. The results are just astounding as their demonstrations seem to show that plants both listen to and create music. They even offer concerts at their community and at festivals worldwide (http://www.damanhur.org/en/research-and-experimentation/the-plant-world)..

I remember attending a private concert given by a friend, a beautiful and sensitive pianist whose work has been featured on national radio in Canada.

She is also a music teacher and prefaced her performance — piano variations of Beethoven — with an explanation of some key musical ideas. Then she launched into the works with a precision of finger movement that caused sounds to float gracefully across the room. I was grateful for her explanations; I could listen to Beethoven with a new understanding. At one point thoughts vanished and there was another level of listening: No words, just sound and silence, sensations of rhythm and emotions being experienced.

After the concert our conversation turned to trees. Since childhood my friend had experienced oneness with trees. About them she spoke haltingly, not sure of the words to use. I was surprised at her hesitation, especially after her elegant exposition of musical ideas, but she explained that earlier in her life she found communication through words immensely difficult, for we do not have the vocabularies for many things that occur within our subjective world. It was not until teaching at university that she discovered she had to use words effectively if she was to help her students.

My friend then told me a story about a forest with beautiful Balsam Poplar that stood behind the house where she once lived.

"I used to play the piano looking across at the Poplar through my window. I was pregnant with my first child and I felt these trees calling to me. This Poplar has a particular sound, a musical rustling that is both incredibly joyful and restless. Every day on seeing this tree there was a sense of jubilation. Their presence conveyed an enthusiasm for living and sense of curiosity. Through these trees I knew perfectly well what kind of child was coming, they even inspired his name."

My friend noted that during illnesses, pregnancy or other poignant experiences one may naturally be open to such states of heightened sensitivity and awareness.

"Those people I shared this experience with may have thought I was a little crazy because I felt that these trees knew I was carrying a child. What happened between the trees and myself wasn't on the level of words, rather there was an exchange of sensation. In the woods I felt my limbs were their branches. It's hard to describe; this feeling was as if I was wearing the trees like a mantle. I was going beyond myself; I was becoming the trees, the wood."

"All through pregnancy they seemed to protect me and through them I would get messages, for example, to be careful about a certain thing. I would know if something was suitable or not in daily life. It was as if the trees were antennas that extended my field of perception. I also felt the trees as very physically grounding; it was a very concrete feeling of presence and alertness, not at all a flighty or ungrounded feeling."

After the birth of her son, the seedlings of the Balsam Poplar seemed to sprout up quickly in the direction of her home, so much so that on a visit the previous owner remarked on how quickly the forest had approached in a few months. Not that my friend made any claims, they might have grown that way anyway, but a little forest of tiny trees arose around where she and her son would sit outside.

Over 20 years later my friend still spoke fondly of these trees. She described her relationship with the Balsam Poplar as having been a privileged release from the burden of words.

"Pass then through this little space of time conformably to nature, and end thy journey in content, just as an olive falls off when it is ripe, blessing nature who produced it, and thanking the tree on which it grew."
—Marcus Aurelius, *Meditations*

"I said that I was a musician, had talked with trees before and gotten music from them. I asked the tree if he would give me his music so I could hear it. It was hard to hear through the stream but I tuned in and could feel the deep note of the trunk of the tree and then the fine, higher vibrations of the branches and, finally, the needles. It was very beautiful, effulgent music as it reached the needles."
—Joel Andrews, harpist, quoted from *Secrets from the Lives of Trees*, Jeffrey Goelitz

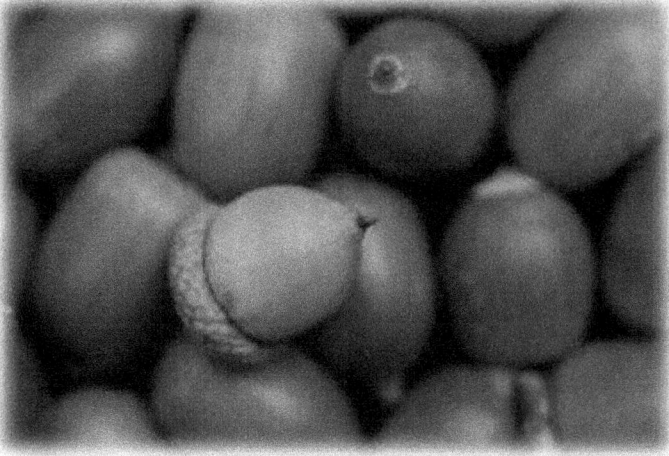

Chapter 24: Feel the Consciousness of a Tree

Daniel Tigner (Hafiz)

"Go to a tree, talk to the tree, touch the tree, embrace the tree, feel the tree. Just sit by the side of the tree, let the tree feel you, that you are a good man and you are not in a mood to harm. By and by friendship arises and you will start feeling that when you come the quality of the tree immediately changes. You will feel it. On the bark of the tree you will feel tremendous energy moving when you come; when you touch the tree she is as happy as a child, as a beloved; when you sit by the tree you will feel many

things. Soon you will be able if you are sad to come to the tree, and just in the presence of the tree your sadness will disappear. Then only will you be able to understand that you are interdependent – you can make the tree happy and the tree can make you happy. And the whole of life is interdependent. This interdependence I call God, Lao Tzu calls Tao – this whole interdependence."
—Osho, *Tao: The Three Treasures, Volume 1*

A Sutras or aphorism describing a meditation technique found in a 5,000 year old Indian Tantra text reads: *"Feel the consciousness of each person as your own consciousness. So, leaving aside concern for self, become each being."*

The mystic Osho suggests first trying this meditation technique with trees because with people it might be difficult in the beginning. Osho says: *"You will be less afraid of a tree so it will be easier. Sitting near a tree, just feel the tree and feel that you have become one with it, that there is a flow within you, a communication, a dialogue, a melting..."*

It is deeply relaxing to put aside all your problems and thoughts for a while and focus on feeling a tree. You are expanding your sense of connectedness and allowing things happening in your life to naturally fall into place. As you get the knack of feeling a tree – its consciousness, how it feels, its life – you open yourself to feeling people in your life much more clearly (and animal friends as well).

How can we approach a tree in order to be with it in such a deep way?

Approach the tree as if it is a valued friend. Be open.

I find it easy to connect by standing tall, my feet solidly on the ground, and using my imagination to feel the roots of the tree and at the same time imagine that my feet are connected to the roots. Then I imagine my legs and torso are merged with the trunk of the tree. My arms reach out in my imagination like the branches. My head and thinking mind are part of the bough of the tree.

Doing this, I am able to rapidly feel a connection, a feeling of strength, grounding and centeredness arising and a quieting of the mind. Not thinking too much and simply being there is what we are gently aiming for, but don't worry or put pressure on yourself if the mind does not seem to slow down.

Every time you do this exercise or meditation, something new may happen, just like when you go out with a human friend and allow yourself to be spontaneous.

Allow yourself to follow your own way of connecting. Be spontaneous. Follow your own inclinations. You might find yourself looking at the beauty of the tree, its physical form, the details of its buds or leaves, or touching its bark and trunk or hugging the tree and feeling its aliveness, its power and grace, even its moods and feelings.

Who knows what might happen if you welcome the tree, and for a time being put aside your human mind - personal thoughts, emotions, feelings or sensations - and simply feel its consciousness. Letting your mind and thought processes become still and fade into the background, allow the consciousness of the tree with its feelings and awareness to arise in you.

In your time together, you might also find yourself talking to the tree about your life, telling the tree about a problem and even asking for its help. A tree is a great listener and being heard is a wonderful healing.

Once your visit is complete, just as with any friend, take some time to say goodbye. Be sure to come back to the present moment, feeling your body, aware of your breathing, aware of any sensations in your human body, so that you are grounded and centered.

A hug and a thank you is always a beautiful way of parting.

Every time you visit, your connection can deepen. As well, overtime, just as when we make a human or animal friend, when we think about them, a certain feeling of them arises, the same can be with a tree. The tree becomes a true friend and part of our inner landscape!

"On the way I stood a moment looking out across the marshes with tall cattails, a patch of water, more marsh, then the woods with a few birch trees shining white at the edge on beyond. In the darkness it all looked just like I felt. Wet and swampy and gloomy, very gloomy. In the morning I painted it. My memory of it is that it was probably my best painting that summer."
—Georgia O'Keeffe

"I wonder what a soul...a person's soul...would look like,' said Priscilla dreamily. 'Like that, I should think,' answered Anne, pointing to a radiance of sifted sunlight streaming through a birch tree. 'Only with shape and features of course. I like to fancy souls as being made of light. And some are all shot through with rosy stains and quivers...and some have a soft glitter like moonlight on the sea...and some are pale and transparent like mist at dawn."
—Lucy Maud Montgomery

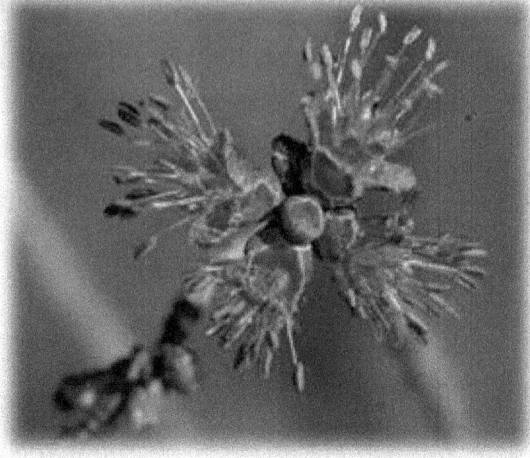

Chapter 25: Biomimicry: Learning from Nature

Kimberly Burnham

Biomimicry or the imitation of life is the process of observing how nature solves challenges and then, implementing similar strategies in our own home, lands, buildings, and materials explains Kimberly Burnham. When you look around at the trees in your yard or your community do they inspire you to create something new or something useful?

What Can We Learn From a Forest?

Some learn to identify
plants trees
and birds

Others the arts
drawing painting
or photography

Still others learn about peace
calmness and spirituality

For some, the forest
is their inspiration
fueling the latest technological advancement

In the natural world
there is no waste
we can learn
from the ultimate recycling center
how to better our own processes

Tree Originated Human Innovations

Velcro
snapped together
by a Swiss engineer
Georges de Mestral
patented nature
burs sticking to his clothes

Design software created
German researcher Claus Mattheck
used in Opel and Mercedes cars
reflect the ways trees and bones
distribute strength
and carry their loads

A fan created by Pax Scientific
borrows from patterns
of swirling kelp
nautilus fractals
and whelks
moving air in an efficient flow

A saltwater-irrigated greenhouse
in the Qatari desert
uses condensation
evaporation tricks

gleaned from the nose of a camel

As redwoods gather fog
India's first hill city
home to more than 300,000
plant deciduous trees
forming a canopy to catch
then reflect through evaporation
a third of the monsoon rain
acting like an engine
driving the monsoon inland
preventing drought

Hydrodynamically efficient shapes
banyan tree leaves mimicked
in water-dispatching roof shingles
water divertment systems
inspired by harvester ants

"Bio-inspired products often see annual doubling in sales when they enter the market. They offer customers better performance, reduced energy requirements, less waste, and less toxicity, while being sold at prices competitive with existing products."
—Jay Harman, *The Shark's Paintbrush: Biomimicry and How Nature is Inspiring Innovation*

What Would Nature Do?

Nature full of clues
climate change can change
we can become producers
of ecosystem services

Translate nature's architecture
engineering strategies
into human design
scaled for our homes

Nature up cycles carbon
harnessing sun power
creating electricity
pumping water

The discovery step
listen to nature
interview the planet's
flora and fauna
30 million living species
only 1.4 million have names

Let's create a Biological Peace Corps
volunteers inventory biodiversity
for two years

we need people who know
all there is in the branches
of nature's tree
immersing ourselves in nature
as we grow from childhood

Echoing nature
with a crossfertilization of ideas
a giant database of biological knowledge
innovation's matchmaker

Stewardship
of wild and settled places
natural outgrowth
of a biomimetic worldview

Nature as a source
of inspiration
mentoring our relationship
with the living world
changes

The only way
to keep learning
safeguard naturalness
the source of all
those good ideas

Two Trees Hold the Other

Struck by beauty
powerful energy
a pair of trees side by side

One Poisonwood Tree
Metopium brownie
with strong bark allergens

The other, a reddish
Gumbo-Limbo tree
Bursera simaruba
contains the poison's antidote

Side by side
they grow
the solution nearby

"Try biomimicry, the discipline of looking to nature for new technologies and designs, to trigger innovative thought."
—David Goldsmith, *Paid to Think: A Leader's Toolkit for Redefining Your Future*

Psychological Mimicry

Take some life coaching from trees ...

"*Never cut a tree down in the wintertime. Never make a negative decision in the low time. Never make your most important decisions when you are in your worst moods. Wait. Be patient. The storm will pass. The spring will come.*"
—Robert H. Schuller

"*Character is like a tree and reputation like a shadow. The shadow is what we think of it; the tree is the real thing.*"
—Abraham Lincoln

"*A people without the knowledge of their past history, origin and culture is like a tree without roots.*"
—Marcus Garvey

"*If you look closely at a tree you'll notice it's knots and dead branches, just like our bodies. What we learn is that beauty and imperfection go together wonderfully.*"
—Matthew Fox

Redwoods in the Fog

Chilean redwood needles
capture desert fog
a unique adaptation
inspiration for technology
bringing much needed water
to the driest areas on the planet

Chile's Atacama Desert
with half an inch of rain
each year
along the coast
the desert has marine fog
mesh nets dubbed "Fog Catchers,"
turn fog into droplets
rolling down into pipes
water collects in tanks
just like in redwood forests

Netting 264 gallons a day
from fog
what will our redwood forests
inspire next...

Tree and Bones Optimize Strength

Wave at trees through your car window
thank them, yes
for your car's crash safety
great gas mileage

Trees engineer themselves
arranging fibers for strength
minimizing stress
like extra padding
beneath a heavy branch

Bones must carry moving loads
shifting material
from not need to needed
optimizing structure
for dynamic load

Car engineers incorporate
lessons learned
trees and bones teach us
new vehicle design
crash tests as safe
30 percent lighter

Plastic "Trees" Convert CO2 into Green Gasoline

Plastic "tree"
designed by lookers of nature
convert atmospheric CO_2
into green gasoline
reuse recycle carbon right out of the air

Improving on nature
plastic trees pull
a thousand times more than Mother Nature
carbon dioxide for cars with green gasoline
captured and sequestered
a quick solution
desperately needed

Climate recovery
a clean energy economy
earth getting hotter
ice caps melting
weather patterns changing
solving the quandary
two scientists inspired by trees invent
plastic trees
for anywhere you want
tomorrow

Nature's math
add hydrogen
capture carbon atoms
re-create gasoline
zero net impact
taking out carbon
burning gasoline put in

Closing the carbon loop
atmospheric carbon converted to gasoline
fuels vehicles without drilling
then collected once again
by "trees" soon to go
from demonstration to deployment

Rooted Like Mangrove Creating Ground

Imagine you're paddling
in a Costa Rican mangrove
your kayak make its way
through tight muddy channels
between rows of tall mangrove trees

Above you the trees spread
their leafy branches
shading you from the sun
keeping the moisture under their leaves

At your sides, a complex network
roots emerge from the waters
a nice habitat for thousands of crabs
and barnacles

Below you, the brown salty waters
move slowly
directions imposed by tide
fresh water from the streams
loaded with sediments
come down the mountain
blends with the salty sea water
here in the mangrove

Red mangrove
a stilt root tree
interconnected tubular arcs
half the network of roots
is in ground
the other half in the sea
conquering new ground

Fascinating strategies
constant tidal exposure
halfway between
salty waters and fresh waters
the ground it sits on
mud

A tree resilient
in a dynamic environment
intricate roots
dive into the water
slow the stream
sediments sink

Think coastal zones
terrain exposed
land sliders take inspiration
constructing on flowing terrains
pontoons house supports

Nature's geometry
straight cylindrical pillars
don't work in unstable zones
use interconnecting arches
structure in different sizes
match pillar density
with roots of a mangrove tree

"Slush is frozen over.
People say that winter lasts forever,
but it's because they obsess
over the thermometer.

North in the mountains,
the maple syrup is trickling.
Brave geese punch through
the thin ice left on the lake.

Underground, pale seeds
roll over in their sleep.
Starting to get restless.
Starting to dream green."
—Laurie Halse Anderson, *Speak*

Bark Cooling

Antibacterial sunscreen bark
keeps surfaces cooling
minimizing solar absorption
heat emissions maximized
physical integrity protect
from abiotic factors

Tree bark optimizes reflectivity
like an optical window
light transmitted
reflected by green vegetation

Tree bark tannins
create optimal radiative temperature
control acting as mediators
excitation energy
photo-antioxidative activity
control of radiation damage

Barks, evolve, adapt, apply
a paper-like structure
sheets peeling off
high heat-insulation
trapping air spaces between them
look at a birch or paper-bark tree

Other barks rough surface
produce shadowed areas
amongst the illuminated ones
cooling the round profile
minimizing the surface to volume
while leaves maximize surface area

*"Biomimicry is basically taking a design challenge and
then finding an ecosystem that's already solved that
challenge, and literally trying to emulate what you learn."*
—Janine Benyus

*"Organisms don't think of CO2
as a poison.*

*Plants and organisms that make
shell,s
coral,
think of it as a building block."*
—Janine Benyus

Flame Retardant Trees

Natural processes offer innovation
the way jack-pine cones open
in the face of heat
to allow reproduction
even as fire destroys the forest

The way eucalyptus trees
shed scattered pieces
of quick-burning bark
to suck up oxygen
and take fire away
from the main trunk

"Life creates conditions
conducive to life."
—Janine Benyus

Sunlight Gathering

Trees follow a mathematical formula
gathering sunlight in crowded forests
we can collect solar energy
in the same way

Fibonacci spirals in plants.
3 5 8 13 21 34 55 around
and round it spirals
bigger and smaller

Repeating patterns
of solar collectors
seed arrangements
and more

*"There are three types of biomimicry - one is copying form
and shape, another is copying a process, like photosynthesis
in a leaf, and the third is mimicking at an ecosystem's level,
like building a nature-inspired city."*
—Janine Benyus

Maple Seed Drone

DARPA's Maple seed inspired drone takes flight
a cue from how maple seed pods drift
long distances using an unusual shape
spiraling themselves
through the air

DARPA's designs a drone
that same spinning motion
to fly
do vertical take-offs

Tricky little maple seed
one wing or two
help it to whirl
in the air as it falls
giving the breeze a chance
to pick it up and carry it
away from the tree

DARPA's drone collect
military intelligence
when tree huggers take over
drones gather data on deforestation
monitoring endangered species
checking in on pollution levels

Spinning on and on
with the lift of air
saving our lives

Lotus = Paint

Sharkskin on dry land
lotus flower's micro-rough surface
sparkles clean
a sea of tiny nail-like protuberances

German Ispo's 4 years observing
brings us a house paint
whose surface pushes away dust and dirt

"The maple tree plays a meaningful role in the historical development of Canada. It contributes to wood products, sustains the maple sugar industry, and beautifies the landscape."
—Planet Collection, *Canada: Picture Book*

"Those who are inspired by a model other than Nature, a mistress above all masters, are laboring in vain."
—Leonardo DaVinci

Oak Tree and Sustainable Architecture

In the face of Hurricane Katrina
ripping through New Orleans
bringing floods and gale-force winds
live oaks are surprisingly resilient
Think like a tree

The tallest living things
leafy towers strategize
protection against threats
solve daunting engineering challenges
think like a tree

The beating a tree gets
from a hurricane's gale force winds
hammering trees with a dynamic blows
unleashing a suite of mechanical problems
the stuff of engineering nightmares
think like a tree

Withstanding high wind speeds
trees deal with wind acceleration
the air's "thrown weight"
its mass, basically
think like a tree

Calms between gusts
can damage too
as the tree rebounds and sways
building up heavy loads on branches and roots
a litany of other factors play
precipitation levels
soil conditions
the state of the surrounding trees
think like a tree

Leaves that work great
for photosynthesizing
a liabilities in high wind
little sails with a lot of drag
release the drag
think like a tree

In 40 mph winds
the leaves of trees
like maple, poplar, and holly
reconfigure into aerodynamic shapes
curling up into little tubes
clumping together into cones
flattening to reduce drag
think like a tree

Strong root systems serve
a countermeasure to the drag
of the leaves
and wind's sideways force
think like a tree

Growing all their own material
takes energy that could be spent
on other needs like reproduction
think like a tree

*"There is something beautiful about all scars of whatever
nature. A scar means the hurt is over, the wound is closed
and healed, done with."*
—Harry Crews

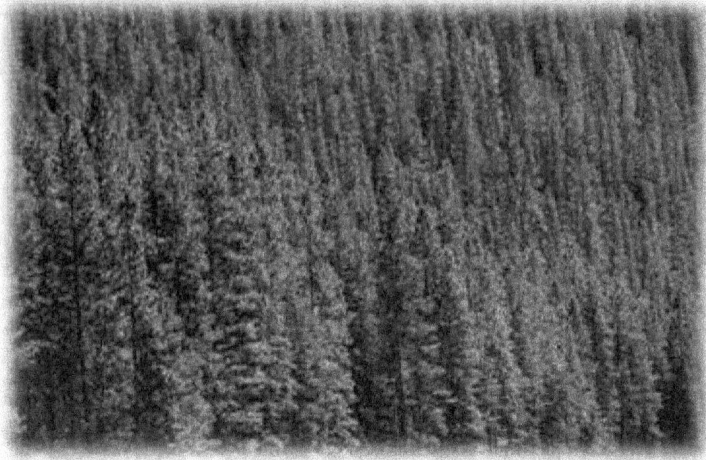

Reading List

Altman, N. (1995). The Deva Handbook: How To Work With Nature's Subtle Energies. Rochester, Vt., Destiny Books.

Andrews, T. (1993). Enchantment Of The Faerie Realm: Communicate With Nature Spirits & Elementals. St. Paul, Minn., U.S.A., Llewellyn Publications.

Arno, S. F. and R. P. Hammerly (2007). Northwest Trees: Identifying And Understanding The Region's Native Trees. Seattle, WA, Mountaineers Books.
    "Finely illustrated and written, both informative and enjoyable."

Arntz, W., B. Chasse, et al. (2005). <u>What The Bleep Do We Know!? Discovering The Endless Possibilities For Altering Your Everyday Reality</u>. Deerfield Beach, Fla., Health Communications.

Backster, C. (2003). <u>Primary Perception: Biocommunication With Plants, Living Foods, And Human Cells</u>. Anza, Calif., White Rose Millennium Press.

Baker, R. S. B. (1949). <u>Green Glory; The Forests Of The World</u>. New York, A.A. Wyn.

Baker, R. S. B. (1959). <u>The Redwoods</u>. London, G. Ronald.
   "Baker contributed to saving the Coastal Redwoods of California, bequeathing something of tremendous beauty to future generations. He is an eloquent writer."

Baker, R. S. B. and Indian National Trust for Art and Cultural Heritage (1989). <u>Richard St. Barbe Baker, Man Of The Trees: A Centenary Tribute</u>. New Delhi, Indian National Trust for Art and Cultural Heritage.

Bloom, W. (2009). <u>Working With Angels, Fairies & Nature Spirits</u>. London, Piatkus.

Boone, J. A. (1954). <u>Kinship With All Life</u>. New York, Harper.

Boone, J. A., P. H. Leonard, et al. (1990). <u>Adventures In Kinship With All Life</u>. Joshua Tree, Calif., Tree of Life Publications.

Bourne, E. J. (2008). <u>Global Shift: How A New Worldview Is Transforming Humanity</u>. Petaluma, CA; Oakland, CA, Noetic Books; New Harbinger Publications.

Boyer, M.-F. (1996). <u>Tree-Talk: Memories, Myths And Timeless Customs</u>. New York, Thames and Hudson.

Bruce, A. (2005). <u>Beyond The Bleep: The Definitive Unathorized Guide To What The Bleep Do We Know!?</u> New York, Disinformation.

Buhner, S. H. (2004). <u>The Secret Teachings Of Plants: The Intelligence Of The Heart In The Direct Perception Of Nature</u>. Rochester, Vt., Bear & Company.

Burnham, K. (1990). "Biological Pest Control: The New Bottom Line, Sparring the Sprayer." <u>The</u>

Growing Edge: Indoor & Outdoor Gardening for Today's High-Tech Grower 1(Winter (2).

Burnham, K. (1990). "Quebec's Hydroponic Tomatoes: An Alternative to European Imports." The Growing Edge: Indoor & Outdoor Gardening for Today's High-Tech Grower 1(Spring (3).

Burnham, K. (2011). Our Fractal Nature, a Journey of Self-Discovery and Connection Psychology Meets Science, The Nerve Whisperer, a Messenger Mini-Book.

"Become empowered by your fractal nature! Our Fractal Nature guides you through concepts and fun exercises to shape your personal healing potential to fit your needs. Tap into fractals to find new energy resources and expand self-awareness. Learn to recognize fractal patterns in your life, select the seed for each beginning, and surf life's rhythms so you can choose to live in a friendly universe!"

Burnham, K. (2011 10 01). Balancing the Sleep-Wake Cycle: Sleep Better, Learn Faster, Contribute More, and Enjoy Life to Its Fullest (Recover Your Life Through Brain Health), Creating Calm Network Publishing Group.

Burnham, K. (2012). Fractals: Seeing the Patterns in Our Existence, a chapter in Jack Canfield's Pearls of Wisdom, 30 inspirational Ideas to Live Your Best Life Now! (April 2, 2012) with 30 authors including CT authors Kimberly Burnham (West Hartford) and Stacy Lee Goforth, (Groton, CT).

Burnham, K. (2012 06 15). Parkinson's Alternatives: Walk Better, Sleep Deeper and Move Consciously; Solutions from Nature's Sensational Medicine.

Burnham, K. (2013). Do You Ever Describe Yourself As Stiff as a Board? Ride-Fit Blog [read more] http://www.ride-fit.com/Blog/Spinning-Bike-And-Turbo-Trainer-Workout-Blog-031113.html.

Burnham, K. and the Poetry Posse (2015). Learning to Heal; What I Learned in the Garden Today; and What I Know (Poetry). Year of the Poet, March 2015 Edition. William S. Peters Sr. New York, NY, Inner Child Press.

Burnham, K. and and the Poetry Posse (2015). My Natural Mind, Summer Rain, Planting Seeds, A Garden Villanelle. New York, NY, Inner Child Press.

Burnham, K., C. M. S. G. Cloutier, et al. (2016). <u>Trees, Healing, and You; Guided Imagery, Poems, Stories, & Other Empowering Tools</u>. Spokane, WA, Creating Calm Network Publishing Group.

Burnham, K., L. Sawyer, et al. (2016). 30 Poems in 30 Days: Writing Prompts & Poems from Tiferet Journal. <u>30 Poems in 30 Days: Writing Prompts & Poems from Tiferet Journal</u>. K. Burnham and L. Sawyer. Creating Calm Network Publishing Group & Tiferet Journal.

Burnham, K., A. White, et al. (2012 11 25). Beyond Seeing and Hearing pg 20. <u>Healing Through Words, Poetry ... Prose ... Prayers ... Stories.</u> The Anthological Writers (Author), William S. Peters Sr. (Designer) New York, New York, Inner Child Press.

Caldecott, M. (1993). <u>Myths Of The Sacred Tree: Including Myths From Africa, Native America, China, Sumeria, Russia, Greece, India, Scandinavia, Europe, Egypt, South America, [And] Arabia</u>. Rochester, Vt.; Colchester, Vt., Destiny Books; Distributed to the book trade in the USA by American International Distribution Corporation (AIDC).

Capra, F. (1996). <u>The Web Of Life: A New Scientific Understanding Of Living Systems</u>. New York, Anchor Books.

Capra, F. (2010). <u>The Tao Of Physics: An Exploration Of The Parallels Between Modern Physics And Eastern Mysticism</u>. Boston, Shambhala.

Carder, A. (1995). <u>Forest Giants of the World - Past and Present.</u> . Markham, Ontario, Canada Fitzhenry & Whiteside
      "A fascinating journey around the world to great trees. A gem of a book."

Chamovitz, D. (2012). <u>What A Plant Knows: A Field Guide To The Senses</u>. New York, Scientific American/Farrar, Straus and Giroux.

Charles, T. Juniper, et al. (2010). <u>Harmony: A New Way Of Looking At Our World</u>. New York, Harper Collins.
      "In this informational, inspirational work, Charles, the Prince of Wales, describes his views on climate change for the first time, presenting a compelling case that the solution to this problem lies in our ability to regain our balance with nature."

Chase, P. and J. Pawlik (1991). <u>Trees For Healing:</u>
<u>Harmonizing With Nature For Personal Growth And</u>
<u>Planetary Balance</u>. North Hollywood, Calif.,
Newcastle.

Chetan, A., D. Brueton, et al. (1994). <u>The Sacred Yew</u>.
London; New York, Arkana.
   "The beautifully written story of the Yew Tree in
the United Kingdom and one man's campaign to preserve
and honor it."

Childre, D. L., H. Martin, et al. (1999). <u>The HeartMath</u>
<u>Solution</u>. San Francisco, CA, HarperSanFrancisco.

Cole, R. V. (1965). <u>The Artistic Anatomy of Trees,</u>
<u>Their Structure & Treatment in Painting</u>. New York,
Dover Publications.
   "A thorough study of the subject and very
interesting."

Conroy, J. and B. Alexander (2011). <u>Tree Whispering:</u>
<u>A Nature Lover's Guide to Touching, Healing, and</u>
<u>Communicating with Trees, Plants, and All of Nature,</u>
Plant Kingdom Communications @
www.PlantKingdomCommunications.com.
   "The book Tree Whispering: A Nature Lover's
Guide to Touching, Healing, and Communicating with

Trees, Plants, and All of Nature offers a simple yet profound and inspiring experience of communicating with Green Beings. It guides readers – step by step and with stories – through conscious practices to come from trees' and plants' point of view. It provides useful bioenergy healing techniques and respectful approaches for rejuvenating tree and plant health from the inside-out while awakening spiritual upliftment. By adopting a wise world-view – moving away from human-centric attitudes and moving toward cooperation, partnership, and co-creativity with all Nature – readers will celebrate their strengthened connections to Nature's Beings."

Conroy, J. and B. Alexander (2012). <u>People Saving Their Trees in Hurricane Sandy</u>, Plant Kingdom Communications

"Enjoy these inspiring, heartfelt, and heroic stories from people who used the Tree Whispering® Storm Prep Whispers™ to help their trees survive Hurricane Sandy and to empower themselves in the face of disaster. "This was one positive thing I could do in the face of feeling so helpless in the storm."–Liz Wassell, Reiki for Animals, New Paltz, New York. "Your Whispers helped me prepare physically, but more importantly, emotionally for the storm, and for the aftermath in my area hit very hard by Hurricane Sandy."–Shelagh W., Mountain Lakes, New Jersey."

Conroy, J. and B. Alexander (2012). <u>Tree Whispering: Trust the Path Notebook and Journal</u>, Plant Kingdom Communications.

"Companion notebook and journal to the book Tree Whispering: A Nature Lover's Guide to Touching, Healing, and Communicating with Trees, Plants, and All of Nature. The companion notebook and journal is small, light-weight and spiral bound for easy opening, carrying, and adding entries. In it, the "Try This" exercises from the book are repeated so that readers may conveniently take it with them anywhere, especially into the woods or out to their backyards, in order to complete the Nature-communication experiences and the practical techniques. The companion notebook and journal also provides space to write personal reflections. The bottom of the journaling pages displays wise quotes and insightful advice from graduates of Tree Whispering workshops."

Conroy, J. and B. Alexander (2013). <u>Messages from Trees: A Coloring Book for the Young and Young-at-Heart</u>, Plant Kingdom Communications.

"The trees are alive—just like you—and have messages for you. If you listen and look with your heart, you'll know what they want to tell you. As you color-in the drawings on these pages, think about what these trees are saying. When you use your crayons, markers, or colored pencils, don't be limited by the lines on the page. You can

add your own ideas. Add different colors. Your pages can look any way you want them to look!"

Conroy, J. and B. Alexander (2013). <u>The Tree Whisperer's 10 Tree and Plant Insights</u>, Plant Kingdom Communications.

"The book Tree Whispering: A Nature Lover's Guide to Touching, Healing, and Communicating with Trees, Plants, and All of Nature offers a simple yet profound and inspiring experience of communicating with Green Beings. It guides readers – step by step and with stories – through conscious practices to come from trees' and plants' point of view. It provides useful bioenergy healing techniques and respectful approaches for rejuvenating tree and plant health from the inside-out while awakening spiritual upliftment. By adopting a wise world-view – moving away from human-centric attitudes and moving toward cooperation, partnership, and co-creativity with all Nature – readers will celebrate their strengthened connections to Nature's Beings."

Conroy, J. and B. Alexander (2014). <u>Live and Let Live: Collaboration Heals Ecosystems</u>, Plant Kingdom Communications.

"The living Beings of Nature want to collaborate with humanity as equals. They want to connect with you and co-create a livable and deeply peaceful world that works

for everyone, including you and them. They want to be partners in humanity's next challenges on Earth: Thriving and prospering while restoring healthy dynamic balance in local and global ecosystems. You are the one they have been waiting for. They want to team up with you. How best can you team up with the living Beings of Nature?

Authoritative and practical must-have tool for an outside-the-box solution to ecosystem degradation. Large-sized book offers large-sized ideas and ingredients for solving humanity's next challenges: Thriving sustainably while restoring healthy interactivity and dynamic balance to ecological systems. Adopt the wise stewardship philosophy of Live-and-Let-Live and use EcoPeace Treaties® for enlightened collaboration with Nature."

Conroy, J. and B. Alexander (2016). <u>Live and Let Live: Enlightened Stewardship</u>, Plant Kingdom Communications.

"Enlightened stewardship of Earth begins with the realization that all who share life on this planet can coexist as interdependent partners. Enlightened stewardship is fulfilled when individuals collaborate with Nature's living Beings in cocreative ways so all can thrive sustainably.

Asking "How can my actions be good for all?" leads to practical changes and personal empowerment. This leading-edge second volume of the Live and Let Live series reveals what's possible for people who learn how to establish a "wanted world" in their backyards and set their minds toward reversing broad ecological damage. All Beings win when ecosystem members regain health.

EcoPeace Treaties® between living Beings and enlightened stewards integrate, harmonize, and bring forth wholes greater than the sum of the parts. Cooperative BioBalance® is a leading-edge area of study and new career field. It examines incorrect assumptions about Nature and is a fresh, intuitive, and grounded new way of implementing wise solutions to environmental issues."

Couplan, F. (1998). The Encyclopedia Of Edible Plants Of North America. New Canaan, Conn., Keats Pub.
    "Comprehensive, with lots of information not seen elsewhere."

Cummings, E. E. and C. Raschka (2001). Little Tree. New York, Hyperion Books For Children.
    "Inspired by a poem by E.E. Cummings, this is the story of a little tree that finds its own special place in the world as a much-loved Christmas tree."

Elias, T. S. (1980). The Complete Trees Of North America: Field Guide And Natural History. New York, Outdoor Life/Nature Books: Van Nostrand Reinhold.

Emoto, M. (2010). Messages From Water And The Universe. Carlsbad, Calif., Hay House.

Emoto, M. and V. Slezak (2006). The Hidden Messages In Water. New York, Simon & Schuster Audio.
    "Using high-speed photography, Dr. Masaru Emoto demonstrates that crystals formed in frozen water reveal changes when specific, concentrated thoughts are directed toward them. Water that flows from clear springs or has been exposed to loving words shows brilliant, complex, and colorful snowflake patterns, while polluted water, or water exposed to negative thoughts, forms incomplete, asymmetrical, dull-colored patterns. Since humans and the earth are composed mostly of water, these findings have profound significance."

Farrar, J. L. and Canadian Forest Service. (1995). Trees in Canada. Ottawa, Fitzhenry & Whiteside Ltd.
    "An authoritative field guide to trees in Canada. A must for the tree lover's library and backpack."

Findhorn Community (1976). The Findhorn Garden. London, Turnstone Books: Wildwood House.

Forsell, M. (1995). The Herbal Grove. New York, Villard Books.

Foster, S. and J. A. Duke (2000). <u>A Field Guide To Medicinal Plants And Herbs Of Eastern And Central North America</u>. Boston, Houghton Mifflin Co.

"Peterson guides are a reliable and user friendly source of information."

Goelitz, J. and S. Royall (1991). <u>Secrets From The Lives Of Trees</u>. Boulder Creek, Calif., Planetary Publications.

"Writing with a charm and innocence. Of note is exploration of the music of trees."

Grescoe, A. (1997). Giants-The Colossal Trees of Pacific North America. Boulder, Colorado, , Robert Rinehart Publishers

"Beautifully photographed and written, a revelation and celebration of the wonder of these giant trees."

Hageneder, F. (2005). <u>The Meaning Of Trees: Botany, History, Healing, Lore</u>. San Francisco, Chronicle Books.

Hawken, P. (2007). <u>Blessed Unrest: How The Largest Movement In The World Came Into Being, And Why No One Saw It Coming</u>. New York, Viking.

Heinrich, B. (1997). <u>The Trees in My Forest</u>. New York, NY, Cliff Street Books

"A lovely and intimate exploration of a forest and its natural history. Science-writing at a very fine level."

Helliwell, T. (1997). <u>Summer With The Leprechauns: A True Story</u>. Nevada City, CA, Blue Dolphin.

Hepper, F. N. (1997). <u>Planting A Bible Garden : A Good Book Practical Guide</u>. Grand Rapids, Mich., F.H. Revell.

Hepper, F. N., C. Molan, et al. (1995). <u>Lands Of The Bible: From Plants And Creatures To Battles And Covenants</u>. Nashville, Tenn., T. Nelson.

Hopman, E. E. (1991). <u>Tree Medicine, Tree Magic</u>. Custer, Wash., Phoenix Pub.

Hora, B. (1981). <u>The Oxford Encyclopedia Of Trees Of The World</u>. Oxford; New York, Oxford University Press.

"Put together by a team of 39 authors. Very informative."

Hunger Project. (1985). <u>Ending Hunger: An Idea Whose Time Has Come</u>. New York, Praeger.

Huntington, H. E. (1962). <u>Forest Giants; The Story Of The California Redwoods</u>. Garden City, N.Y., Doubleday.

Jorgenson, L. (1992). <u>Grand Trees Of America: Our State And Champion Trees</u>. Niwot, Colo., Roberts Rinehart Publishers.

Kaplan, A. (1985). <u>Jewish Meditation: A Practical Guide</u>. New York, Schocken Books.

Kaza, S. (1993). <u>The Attentive Heart: Conversations With Trees</u>. New York, Fawcett Columbine.
    "A fine work of contemplative writing — honest, poetic and insightful."

Kelly, P. (1997). <u>The Elves Of Lily Hill Farm: A Partnership With Nature</u>. St. Paul, Minn., Llewellyn Publications.

Krishnamurti, J. (1993). <u>Krishnamurti To Himself: His Last Journal</u>. San Francisco, HarperSanFrancisco.
    "Krishnamurti is such a wonderful observer!"

Krishnamurti, J. and E. Blau (2002). <u>Meditations</u>. Boston; New York, Shambhala; Distributed in the United States by Random House.

Lappé, F. M. (2011). Ecomind: Changing The Way We Think, To Create The World We Want. New York, Nation Books.

Laszlo, E. and K. Dennis (2013). Dawn Of The Akashic Age: New Consciousness, Quantum Resonance, And The Future Of The World.
"A preview of the post-mechanistic, holistic world in 2020 and 2030 as well as a map of the obstacles we must overcome to get there"

Lewington, A. and E. Parker (1999). Ancient Trees Trees That Live For 1000 Years. London; New York, Collins & Brown; Distributed in the U.S. and Canada by Sterling Pub. Co.

Lippe-Biesterfeld, I. v. and J. v. Tijn (2005). Science, Soul, And The Spirit Of Nature: Leading Thinkers On The Restoration Of Man And Creation. Rochester, Vt., Bear & Co.

Lipton, B. H. (2008). The Biology Of Belief: Unleashing The Power Of Consciousness, Matter & Miracles. Carlsbad, Calif., Hay House.
"Author Lipton is a former medical school professor and research scientist. His experiments, and those of other leading-edge scientists, have examined in great detail the

processes by which cells receive information. The implications of this research radically change our understanding of life. It shows that genes and DNA do not control our biology; that instead DNA is controlled by signals from outside the cell, including the energetic messages emanating from our positive and negative thoughts. Dr. Lipton's profoundly hopeful synthesis of the latest and best research in cell biology and quantum physics is being hailed as a breakthrough, showing that our bodies can be changed as we retrain our thinking."

Little, C. E. (1995). The Dying Of The Trees: The Pandemic In America's Forests. New York, N.Y., Viking.

Lovelock, J. (2000). Gaia: A New Look At Life On Earth. Oxford ; New York, Oxford University Press.

Maclean, D. (2004). Seeds Of Inspiration: Deva Flower Messages. Issaquah, WA, Lorian Association.

Maclean, D. (2006). Call Of The Trees. Issaquah, WA, Lorian Association.

Mason, F. (1972). The Great Design; Order And Progress In Nature. Freeport, N.Y.,, Books for Libraries Press.

Mayor, D. F. and M. S. Micozzi (2011). Energy Medicine East And West: A Natural History Of Qi. Edinburgh; New York, Churchill Livingstone/Elsevier.

McTaggart, L. (2002). The Field: The Quest For The Secret Force Of The Universe. New York, NY, HarperCollins.

McTaggart, L. (2008). The Intention Experiment: Using Your Thoughts To Change Your Life And The World. New York, Free Press.

Medsger, O. P. (1939). Edible Wild Plants. New York,, The Macmillan company.

Menninger, E. A. (1995). Fantastic Trees. Portland, Or., Timber Press.
    "A look at fantastic trees from around the world."

Meyer, J. G. and S. Linnea (2001). America's Famous And Historic Trees: From George Washington's Tulip Poplar To Elvis Presley's Pin Oak. Boston, Houghton Mifflin.

Miller, D. S. and S. Schuett (2002). Are Trees Alive? New York, Walker.

"An introduction to trees that compares parts of a tree to parts of the human body, with illustrations and brief descriptions of trees found around the world."

Mitchell, A. F. and D. More (1987). The Trees Of North America. New York, NY, Facts On File Publications.

Morton, B. R. (1949). Native Trees Of Canada. Ottawa, Dept. of Mines and Resources, Mines, Forests and Scientific Services Branch.
    "An older but still very fine guidebook."

Muir, J. and M. P. Branch (2001). John Muir's Last Journey: South To The Amazon And East To Africa: Unpublished Journals And Selected Correspondence. Washington, Island Press/Shearwater Books.

Muir, J. and F. D. White (2006). Essential Muir. Santa Clara, Calif.; Berkeley, Calif., Santa Clara University; Heyday Books.
    "Like Muir himself, Essential Muir packs an astounding range of experience into a lithe frame: ecstatic yet scientific descriptions of Yosemite; the heartrending tale of that "wee, hairy, sleekit beastie," Stickeen; reflections on the society of Eskimos; Muir's touching tribute, after a lifetime of wonder, to the mighty baobob trees of Africa; and

more. Fred D. White's selection from Muir's writings, and his illuminating commentary, reveal the coherence and drama of a remarkable life: new readers will understand why Muir has become an American icon, and readers who are familiar with his work will be delighted with this fresh look. Muir's fierce love of all of nature, from squirrels to glaciers (but perhaps not sheep), continues to inspire us nearly a century after his death."

Narby, J. (2005). <u>Intelligence In Nature: An Inquiry Into Knowledge</u>. New York, Jeremy P. Tarcher/Penguin.

Oschman, J. L. (2003). <u>Energy Medicine In Therapeutics And Human Performance</u>. Amsterdam ; Boston, Butterworth Heinemann.

Osho <u>Mindfulness In The Modern World: How Do I Make Meditation Part Of Everyday Life?</u>

Osho (1993). <u>The Everyday Meditator</u>. Rutland, Vermont, Charles E. Tuttle, Bibliography and Resources Company.
   "A wonderful resource book for anyone journeying into meditation. A treasure trove of meditations for everyday life including a number of tree meditations."

Osho (1994). <u>From Medication to Meditation</u>. Saffron Walden, C. W. Daniel.
"The role of meditation in healing."

Osho (2010). <u>The Book of Secrets: 112 Meditations to Discover the Mystery Within: an Introduction to Meditation</u>. New York, St. Martin's Press.
"Covering the 112 seed Meditation of Tantra: it is an invaluable source of insight for all meditators."

Pakenham, T. (1996). <u>Meetings With Remarkable Trees</u>. London, Weidenfeld & Nicolson.

Pearlman, N. and Educational Communications Collection (Library of Congress) (1991). <u>Econews. A Look At: Man Of The Trees—Richard St. Barbe Baker</u>. United States, Educational Communications, Inc.

Peattie, D. C. (2007). <u>A Natural History Of North American Trees</u>. Boston, Houghton Mifflin.

Peattie, D. C. and P. Landacre (1991). <u>A Natural History Of Western Trees</u>. Boston, Houghton Mifflin Co.

Perlin, J. (1991). A Forest Journey: The Role Of Wood In The Development Of Civilization. Cambridge, Mass., Harvard University Press.

Phillips, R. and S. Grant (1978). Trees of North America and Europe. New York, Random House.

Phillips, R. and M. Rix (1989). The Random House Book of Shrubs. New York, Random House.

Platt, R. H. (1965). The Great American Forest. Englewood Cliffs, N.J., Prentice-Hall.

Platt, R. H. (1992). 1001 Questions Answered About Trees. New York, Dover Publications.

Pogacnik, M. (2010). Nature Spirits & Elemental Beings: Working with the Intelligence in Nature.

Pollan, M. (2001). The Botany Of Desire: A Plant's Eye View Of The World. New York, Random House.

Pollan, S. M. and M. Levine (2003). Second Acts: Creating The Life You Really Want, Building The Career You Truly Desire. New York, HarperResource.

Ramana, A., edited with additional writing by Daniel Tigner, (2016). <u>American Mystic: Memoirs of a Happy Man</u>, Inquiry Books

"*About A. Ramana's life and awakening as recounted to Saroja G. Poilblan*"

Raven, P. H., R. F. Evert, et al. (2013). <u>Biology of Plants</u>. New York, W.H. Freeman and Company Publishers.

Rhoads, A. F. and T. A. Block (2007). <u>The Plants Of Pennsylvania: An Illustrated Manual</u>. Philadelphia, University of Pennsylvania Press.

"*A very thorough and meticulous reference to plants in Pennsylvania, and also a very helpful reference to plants of the Northeast.*"

Ribner, M. (1998). <u>Everyday Kabbalah: A Practical Guide To Jewish Meditation, Healing And Personal Growth</u>. Secaucus, NJ, Carol Pub. Group.

Riddell, C. (1991). <u>The Findhorn Community: Creating A Human Identity For The 21st Century</u>. Findhorn, Forres, Moray, Scotland, Findhorn Press.

Roads, M. J. (1987). Talking With Nature: Sharing The Energies And Spirit Of Trees, Plants, Birds, And Earth. Tiburon, Calif., H.J. Kramer.

Rokach, A. and A. Millman (1995). The Field Guide to Photographing Trees. New York, Amphoto Books.
"Although it is about film photography, the underlying principles of capturing a beautiful image of a tree still apply."

Russell, P. (2007). The Global Brain: The Awakening Earth In A New Century. Edinburgh, Floris Books.

Sale, E. V. (1978). Quest For The Kauri: Forest Giants And Where To Find Them. Wellington, Reed.

Sandell, R., J. Dodd, et al. (2010). Re-Presenting Disability: Activism And Agency In The Museum. London ; New York, Routledge.

Sandved, K. B., G. T. Prance, et al. (1993). Bark: The Formation, Characteristics, And Uses Of Bark Around The World. Portland, Or., Timber Press.
"Fascinating and wonderful photography by Kjell B. Sandved of the Smithsonian Institute."

Schneck, M. and K. p. Burnham (1990). <u>Butterflies—How To Identify And Attract Them To Your Garden</u>. Emmaus, Pa.; New York, N.Y., Rodale Press; Distributed in the book trade by St. Martin's Press.

Schneck, M. and K. p. Burnham (1992). Gardening in Small Spaces (Hardcover) Smithmark Publishers Inc. / Quintet Publishing Limitied, A Quintet Book / Central Southern Typesetters / Start Standard Industries Private Ltd.: 80 pages.

Schwartz, G. E. and W. L. Simon (2007). <u>The Energy Healing Experiments: Science Reveals Our Natural Power To Heal</u>. New York, Atria Books.

Seuss (1974). <u>The Lorax, and Horton Hears a Who, Dr. Seuss Storytime</u>. New York, Random House.

Seuss, J. Schulman, et al. (2004). <u>Your Favorite Seuss: 13 Stories Written And Illustrated By Dr. Seuss With 13 Introductory Essays</u>. New York, Random House Children's Books.
    "A compilation of more than a dozen previously published Dr. Seuss books, plus essays by nine authors and other book lovers, including Audrey Geisel, widow of Dr. Seuss."

Shapton, L. (2010). The Native Trees Of Canada. Montreal; New York, Drawn & Quarterly Pub; Distributed in the USA by Farrar, Straus and Giroux.

Shaw, J. (1994). John Shaw's Landscape Photography. New York, Amphoto.

Sheldrake, R. (1994). The Rebirth Of Nature: The Greening Of Science And God. Rochester, Vt., Park Street Press.

Soper, J. H. and M. L. Heimburger (1982). Shrubs of Ontario. Toronto, ROM.
"A comprehensive field guide that can help with identification of shrubs not only in Ontario but the adjacent Northern States and Quebec."

Stewart, H. (1984). Cedar: Tree of Life to the Northwest Coast Indians. Vancouver, B.C.; Seattle, WA, Douglas & McIntyre; University of Washington Press.
"Learn about the place of Yellow Cedar and Red Cedar in Northwest Native societies."

Symonds, G. W. D. (1958). The Tree Identification Book: A New Method For The Practical Identification And Recognition Of Trees. New York, M. Barrows.

Symonds, G. W. D. (1963). <u>The Shrub Identification Book; The Visual Method For The Practical Identification Of Shrubs, Including Woody Vines And Ground Covers</u>. New York, M. Barrows.

> *"Both of Symonds books are a great help in the identification of trees and shrubs."*

Thomas, L. and C. Obry (2010). <u>The Encyclopedia Of Energy Medicine</u>. Minneapolis, Minn., Fairview Press.

Tigner, D. (1990). <u>The Art of Grant Tigner (Daniel's father)</u>.

Tigner, D. (1998). <u>Canadian Forest Tree Essences – Healing Through the Natural Resonance of Trees</u>.

Tigner, D., C. Cloutier, et al. (2013). <u>Trees Speak – Vibrational Tree Essences Guidebook</u>.

Tigner, D. and G. L. Jabour (2014). <u>The Time of Your Life – Everyone Has a Story (about the wisdom journeys of 40 people aged 50 and over)</u>, Revealing Light Productions.

Tigner, D. and J. Sutton (2015). <u>Sam and the Sea Monsters (a sports story for girls from 9 to 15)</u>.

Tompkins, P. and H. Rudd (1973). The Secret Life Of Plants. Vital history cassettes no. 1 for Dec. 73. New York, Encyclopedia Americana/CBS News Audio Resource Library,

"Author Peter Tompkins discusses his contention in his book, The secret life of plants, that plants react to outside stimuli, people, places, everything."

Tudge, C. (2005). The Secret Life Of Trees. London; New York, Allen Lane.

Turner, N. J. and A. F. Szczawinski (1979). Edible Wild Fruits and Nuts Of Canada. Ottawa, National Museum of Natural Sciences.

"Contains many good recipes worthwhile trying."

Van Pelt, R. Forest Giants Of The Pacific Coast. Vancouver; San Francisco, Global Forest Society in association with University of Washington Press.

Watts, A. (1972). The Book; On The Taboo Against Knowing Who You Are. New York, Vintage Books.

West, D. (2012). Cetiosaurus and Other Dinosaurs and Reptiles From The Middle Jurassic. New York, Gareth Stevens Pub.

Wilber, K. (1999). <u>The Collected Works Of Ken Wilber</u>. Boston, Shambhala.

Wilber, K. (2000). <u>A Brief History Of Everything</u>. Boston; New York, Shambhala; Distributed in the United States by Random House.

Winter, J. (2008). <u>Wangari's Trees Of Peace: A True Story From Africa</u>. Orlando Fla., Harcourt.
"This true story of Wangari Maathai, environmentalist and winner of the Nobel Peace Prize, is a shining example of how one woman's passion, vision, and determination inspired great change."

Wright, M. S. (1997). <u>Behaving As If The God In All Life Mattered</u>. Jeffersonton, Va., Perelandra.

Wright, M. S. (2012). <u>The Perelandra Garden Workbook</u>. Jeffersonton, VA, Perelandra, Ltd.

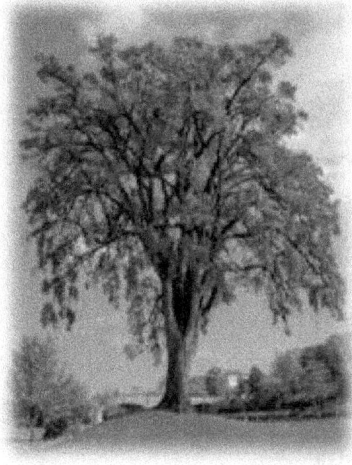

List of Photographs

Cover photo, "Meditation in Old Growth Forest", photo courtesy Daniel Tigner ©2016.

p. 15, "White Spruce (*Picea glauca*)", photo courtesy Daniel Tigner ©2016.

p. 17, "Sugar Maple (*Acer saccharum*) leaves Against Sky", photo courtesy Daniel Tigner ©2016.

p. 21, "Trees on Snowy Hills, Alberta", photo courtesy Daniel Tigner ©2016.

p. 43, "Sugar Maple (*Acer saccharum*) in a Field", photo courtesy Daniel Tigner ©2016.

p. 68, "Gulabo beneath Californian Live Oak", photo courtesy Daniel Tigner ©2016.

p. 75, "Trees-White Spruce (Picea glauca) and Marsh", photo courtesy Daniel Tigner ©2016.

p. 87, "Eastern White Pine (*Pinus strobus*) Needles", photo courtesy Daniel Tigner ©2016.

p. 92, "White Oak in Winter", photo courtesy Daniel Tigner ©2016.

p. 101, "Beech Tree (*Fagus grandifolia*) Looking Up", photo courtesy Daniel Tigner ©2016.

p. 112, "Snowshoeing in Quebec, Canada", photo courtesy Daniel Tigner ©2016.

p. 117, "Resting Beneath a Pine", photo courtesy Daniel Tigner ©2016.

p. 133, "Tree Profile at Dusk in California", photo courtesy Daniel Tigner ©2016.

p. 166, "Woman along Fall Path", photo courtesy Daniel Tigner ©2016.

p. 190, "Mock Orange (*Philadelphus sp.*) Flowers", photo courtesy Daniel Tigner ©2016.

p. 198, "Trees and Hills, California", photo courtesy Daniel Tigner ©2016.

p. 201, "Bitternut Hickory (*Carya cordiformis*) in Spring Woods", photo courtesy Daniel Tigner ©2016.

p. 214, "Forest and Mountains", photo courtesy Daniel Tigner ©2016.

p. 229, "Céline and Jason Examining a Juniper", photo courtesy Daniel Tigner ©2016.

p. 237, "Great White Elm (*Ulmus americana*)", photo courtesy Daniel Tigner ©2016.

p. 247, "Red Oak (*Quercus rubra*) Spring Catkins", photo courtesy Daniel Tigner ©2016.

p. 305, "Winter by Lake Superior", photo courtesy Daniel Tigner ©2016.

p. 310, "Bark of Silver Maple (*Acer saccharinum*)", photo courtesy Daniel Tigner ©2016.

p. 315 "Leaves and Acorns, White Oak (*Quercus alba*)", photo courtesy Daniel Tigner ©2016.

p. 318 "Giant Sequoia (*Sequoiadendron giganteum*) », photo courtesy Daniel Tigner ©2016.

p. 323, "Acorns, Red Oak (*Quercus rubra*)", photo courtesy Daniel Tigner ©2016.

p. 328, "Flower of Red Maple (*Acer rubrum*)", photo courtesy Daniel Tigner ©2016.

p. 352, "Alberta's Western Forest", photo courtesy Daniel Tigner ©2016.

p. 383, "Ottawa Great Elm", photo courtesy Daniel Tigner ©2016.

p. 386, "Trembling Aspen", photo courtesy Daniel Tigner ©2016.

p. 395, "Vancouver Island Trees", photo courtesy Daniel Tigner ©2016.

Author's Biographies

Kimberly Burnham

Life spirals. As a 28-year-old photographer, Kimberly Burnham appreciated beauty. Then an ophthalmologist diagnosed her with a genetic eye condition saying, "Consider what your life will be like if you become blind." Devastating words trickling down into her soul, she discovered a healing path with insight, magnificence, and vision. Today, a poet and neurosciences expert with a PhD in Integrative Medicine, Kimberly's life mission is to change the face of global brain health. Using health coaching, poetry, Reiki, Matrix Energetics, craniosacral therapy, acupressure, and energy medicine, she supports people in their healing from brain, nervous system, chronic pain, and eyesight issues.

In 2013 at age 56, her vision better than when she was 40, Kimberly bicycled over 3000 miles across the US with Hazon in support of sustainable agriculture and food justice.

Kimberly has contributed prose, poetry, and photographs to over 70 books available on Amazon.

Contact her for health coaching and brain health solutions: www.NerveWhisperer.com (860) 221-8510 or NerveWhisperer@gmail.com

Céline Cloutier (Gulabo)

Céline Cloutier - Increasing Your Vibrational Frequency Naturally! *Her meditation name from Osho is Ma Sundar Gulabo, meaning "beautiful rose." Céline Cloutier has been described as "a beautiful soul with a mission of sharing the gifts of our native forests." Her work is both with tree essences – she is co-creator of Canadian Forest Tree Essences – and with people's essences.

"You are wholeness, you are pure love, you deserve it all, and that is your birthright!" Céline writes. And, she's not speaking of a theory or a nice idea, because in 1999 she had a transformative awakening experience that brought her to the pure source of consciousness. She shares that story for the first time in this book out of the knowing that this awakening is available to anyone reading these words.

Some biographical highlights about Céline Cloutier:
*She lives in the wonderful French speaking province of Quebec, Canada.
*She is President of Canadian Forest Tree Essences.
*Her university studies were in dance and psychology.

*Her tall, handsome, kind, brilliant son, Jason, is an architect.

*She has special training as a mediator and in conflict resolution.

*She was director for several years of a Waldorf school and taught kindergarten there.

*She delights in helping people unblock and discover the path to their own essence.

*She is passionate about trees and sharing their healing energies through tree essences!

Learn more about Céline and her work with tree essences at www.essences.ca. To contact Céline Cloutier: Email: Gulabo@essences.ca

Telephone (819) 319-6162

Daniel Tigner (Hafiz)

Daniel Tigner (aka Swami Nirava Hafiz) – Feeling the Consciousness of Trees!

Friends say that Daniel is loving, generous, open hearted to all mankind, and in tune and harmony with the gifts of what nature has to offer. His life is about making the world a better place and sharing with all consciousness, meditation, healing, and knowledge.

The ancient meditation practice of feeling the consciousness of another being is at the core of Daniel's approach to working with trees, whether developing vibrational tree essences in the lineage of Bach Flower Remedies (Canadian Forest Tree Essences), writing about trees, creating a library of images of over 3,000 species of plants or exploring tree meditations described in this book.

"I love communing with trees and discovering their healing and energy properties. I am fascinated by the question of how we can get to know these wonderful living presences, not just from the outside, but directly, as fellow travelers on this planet."

*Daniel has a graduate degree in education in English and Moral Education, and teaches English as a Second Language at the college level.

*Spent 2 years in the Osho International Commune in Pune, India working and meditating.

*Recently circumambulated the sacred mountain of Shiva, Arunachala, in Tiruvannamalai, Southern India on a trip to do research for the book *American Mystic: Memoirs of a Happy Man* (2016).

*Daniel teaches meditation and coaches those on the path of enlightenment and shares with anyone interested in questions related to healing and health.

Learn more about Daniel and his work with trees, writing and photography at www.revealinglightproductions.com and www.essences.ca.

Contact Daniel Tigner @ daniel@danieltigner.com and (819)-682-0205

Margo Royce

* Founder and President: Spirit Inc.
* Co-Founder and First President: The Company of Musical Theatre
* Founder, Director, Producer, Choreographer and Script Writer: The Company of Young Canadians
* Author of Yes You Can! and with a long list of published and performance credits
* Writer and Photographer with artistic group representing Canada in China
* Project Manager of many large national and international projects for clients including: Bank of Canada, NAV CANADA and Portrait Gallery of Canada

Whether as a professional dancer, choreographer, teacher, fitness specialist and all of the above, Margo has touched and been deeply touched by, the many people, environments and creatures who have shared with her, this journey of life. They have all made a lasting and positive difference upon each other.

To contact Margo: spirit@travel-net.com

Jim Conroy and Basia Alexander

Jim Conroy, PhD., and Ms. Basia Alexander are co-founders of the Institute for Cooperative BioBalance, co-authors of 7 books, and co-creators of the Tree Whispering®, Cooperative BioBalance®, and Eco-Peace Treaty® systems for tree, plant, and ecosystem bioenergy healing.

Dr. Conroy received his PhD. in Plant Pathology from Purdue University, left a successful career in the ag-chem industry after an epiphany to become The Tree Whisperer® and an expert Nature Communicator™. Research using his multidimensional model is cutting edge. He is an impassioned speaker and ingenious visionary for collaboration with Nature, including invasive organisms.

Ms. Alexander invents new systems that catalyze transformation in human consciousness. As a future-seeing culture shifter she writes, publishes, and speaks about conscious co-creativity, practical spirituality, health, nature-based communication, and her original insights into the elemental world's structure.

www.TreeWhispering.com
www.CooperativeBioBalance.org

www.EcoPeaceTreaties.org
www.TheTreeWhisperer.com
www.TreeProtector.org
www.PlantKingdomCommunications.com

Ms. Basia Alexander
Co-Founder, Institute for Cooperative BioBalance
Co-Author of 7 books
201-745-5494
www.CooperativeBioBalance.org
https://www.facebook.com/Cooperative-BioBalance-Tree-Whispering-275684945860235/

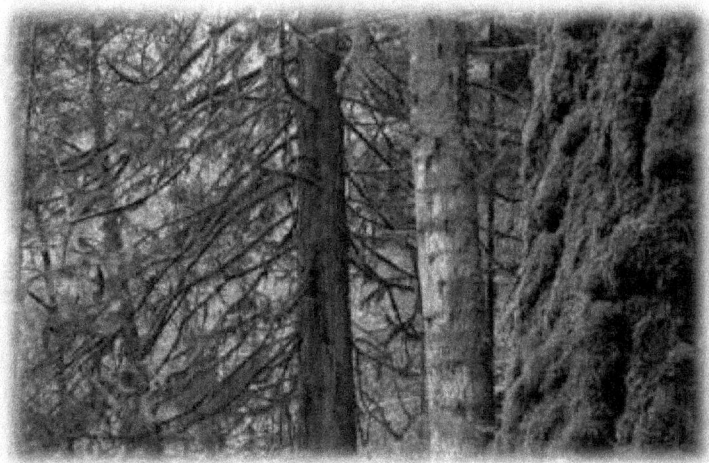

Index

Paterson, Jacqueline
Memory, 244

pectoralis major
(shoulder muscle), 27

pericardium, 29

Pine, 38, 49, 128, 167,
168, 169, 170, 171,
189, 300, 309, 345, 384

Pinenuts, 206

Plath, Sylvia, 53

Pollan, Michael, 56

pomegranates, 29

Poplar, 298, 311, 320,
322, 350

prana, 103

Press, Althea, 203, 205

Proust, Marcel, 175

Quantum physics, 119

Ramana, 93, 129, 130,
376

Reagan, Ronald, 67

red, 29, 30, 73, 88, 89,
90, 100, 168, 187, 311,
341

relaxation, 32, 99, 145

Renterghem, Tony van,
106

Resinies, 209

Rilke, Rainer Maria, 39,
104

River Birches, 70

Rocco, Alicia, 95

Ronald, R.D., 228

Rootie Personalities,
202, 210

Roots, 196, 200, 238,
272

Rouault, Gerorges, 54

Rowling, J. K., 39

Royce, Margo, 1, 2, 15,
133, 166, 392

Rubin, Marty, 276

Rumi, 181, 195

Sacred Grove, 113

Sagan, Carl, 59

Sagarpriya, Ma, 219

Schuller, Robert H., 335

Schulz, Charles M., 284

Schwartz, Stuart, 241

Schweitzer, Albert, 166

Seedie Personalities,
202, 211

Sequoia, 385

Shadyac, Tom, 267

Shakespeare, William,
51, 118

Sheldrake, Rupert, 19

silver, 26

Simard, Professor, 237,
238

sleep, 32, 152, 217

small intestine, 29

www.ingramcontent.com/pod-product-compliance
Lightning Source LLC
Chambersburg PA
CBHW050449270326
41927CB00009B/1667